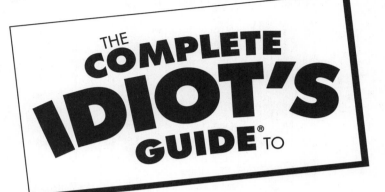

THE COMPLETE IDIOT'S GUIDE TO

Secrets of Longevity

*by Kandeel Judge, M.D.,
and Maxine Barish-Wreden, M.D.,
with Karen K. Brees, Ph.D.*

ALPHA

A member of Penguin Group (USA) Inc.

This book is dedicated to our teachers: our families, our patients, and our readers. We wish you true healing and longevity of mind, body, and spirit.

ALPHA BOOKS

Published by the Penguin Group

Penguin Group (USA) Inc., 375 Hudson Street, New York, New York 10014, USA

Penguin Group (Canada), 90 Eglinton Avenue East, Suite 700, Toronto, Ontario M4P 2Y3, Canada (a division of Pearson Penguin Canada Inc.)

Penguin Books Ltd., 80 Strand, London WC2R 0RL, England

Penguin Ireland, 25 St. Stephen's Green, Dublin 2, Ireland (a division of Penguin Books Ltd.)

Penguin Group (Australia), 250 Camberwell Road, Camberwell, Victoria 3124, Australia (a division of Pearson Australia Group Pty. Ltd.)

Penguin Books India Pvt. Ltd., 11 Community Centre, Panchsheel Park, New Delhi—110 017, India

Penguin Group (NZ), 67 Apollo Drive, Rosedale, North Shore, Auckland 1311, New Zealand (a division of Pearson New Zealand Ltd.)

Penguin Books (South Africa) (Pty.) Ltd., 24 Sturdee Avenue, Rosebank, Johannesburg 2196, South Africa

Penguin Books Ltd., Registered Offices: 80 Strand, London WC2R 0RL, England

Copyright © 2008 by Kandeel Judge and Maxine Barish-Wreden

International Standard Book Number: 978-1-59257-740-8
Library of Congress Catalog Card Number: 2008927333

10 09 08   8 7 6 5 4 3 2 1

Interpretation of the printing code: The rightmost number of the first series of numbers is the year of the book's printing; the rightmost number of the second series of numbers is the number of the book's printing. For example, a printing code of 08-1 shows that the first printing occurred in 2008.

Printed in the United States of America

Note: This publication contains the opinions and ideas of its authors. It is intended to provide helpful and informative material on the subject matter covered. It is sold with the understanding that the authors and publisher are not engaged in rendering professional services in the book. If the reader requires personal assistance or advice, a competent professional should be consulted.

The authors and publisher specifically disclaim any responsibility for any liability, loss, or risk, personal or otherwise, which is incurred as a consequence, directly or indirectly, of the use and application of any of the contents of this book.

Most Alpha books are available at special quantity discounts for bulk purchases for sales promotions, premiums, fund-raising, or educational use. Special books, or book excerpts, can also be created to fit specific needs.

For details, write: Special Markets, Alpha Books, 375 Hudson Street, New York, NY 10014.

Publisher: *Marie Butler-Knight*
Editorial Director: *Mike Sanders*
Senior Managing Editor: *Billy Fields*
Senior Acquisitions Editor: *Paul Dinas*
Development Editor: *Lynn Northrup*
Production Editor: *Kayla Dugger*
Copy Editor: *Cate Schwenk*

Cartoonist: *Steve Barr*
Cover Designer: *Bill Thomas*
Book Designer: *Trina Wurst*
Indexer: *Angie Bess*
Layout: *Brian Massey*
Proofreader: *John Etchison*

Contents at a Glance

Contents

Foreword

The secret to longevity is not to be found simply in the mechanistic, technological world of supplements and medications. When we do not see the total picture in our quest for immortality, we pray at the altar of modern medicine to heal us, and our quest for longevity becomes just another chapter in the frenetic pace of our modern life. We learn to take herbs, supplements, prescriptions, and vitamins. We rush for the latest and newest tests and remedies and technologies. Suffice it to say, there is a lot that modern medicine has to offer, especially in the curing realm. Our average life span has increased from 50 years to over 75 years in the last century alone. Much of that is due to advancements in science and medical care, but why are we insisting on the newest technology when, at the same time, we are obese, addicted to destructive behavior and substances, and self-destructive in so many ways?

A good life is more than just a collection of many days or years on this earth, isn't it? What most of us are really seeking is some kind of purpose, a way in which our unique contribution to the world is made manifest, a way in which to deeply connect with others and ultimately to know that we are loved and that we make a difference. And this, my friends, is the most important secret to a great life: living every day and every moment being the gift that you are (knowing that it might be your last or your loved one's last); bringing to it all of the love and commitment you can muster; and knowing that when your time here on earth has come to an end, you will have been richly satisfied with the journey. By doing this you do not lose your life, but rather, you create it.

Curing diseases and healing lives are two very separate entities. It is easier to take a pill than to change one's life. Health care practitioners need to realize the importance of self-love and self-esteem. We know from studies that those who grow up feeling unloved seek physical and emotional pleasure in drugs, alcohol, food, and behavior that puts their health and their lives at risk. This book is not about guilt, blame and shame, and what you did wrong. This book was written to help you redirect your lives physically, emotionally, and spiritually. If you have lost your health, this book can help you find it once again.

Life is a labor pain of self-creation and growth, and Dr. Max and Dr. Kay are here to be your midwives to a new life. Do you want to live to be 100? If your answer to the question is yes, read on. Our lives are stored within us. We see this when we transplant organs and memories go with them. For us to live a long and richly satisfying life, we have to focus on healing and reconnecting with parts of our bodies and our lives we may have forgotten, or perhaps never considered integral to our longevity.

We have to remember who we are, how precious we are, and how much our lives are a gift. In that reconnection, not only are we more able to give and receive love, but we are also compelled to take care of our physical bodies, as well as the earth, with more reverence.

I have said in the past that body and mind is a unit, bound together via nerve and messenger molecules. Because of this, all healing is self-induced. The new science of psychoneuroimmunology is confirming what many of us have known on a gut level all along: love, hope, joy, and peace of mind have physiological consequences, just as depression and despair do.

We need one another to heal. Loving relationships enhance our health and prolong our lives, as do optimism, hope, joy, a sense of humor, forgiveness, and gratitude. It is vital that we keep that inner child alive and cultivate a childlike sense of humor that can help us survive difficult times.

In *The Complete Idiot's Guide to Secrets of Longevity*, Dr. Max and Dr. Kay have laid out a comprehensive and unique approach to longevity. Using their combined experience as actively practicing internal medicine physicians, they have provided a concise and clear summary of medical factors that impact longevity. They have provided guidelines to staying abreast of the latest medical care that can prolong your life. They have outlined clear recommendations for avoiding the most common diseases likely to reduce your quality of life, impact your longevity, and shorten your life span.

I highly recommend that you read this book, not only to learn what modern medicine has to offer in your quest for longevity, but more importantly, to learn how to cultivate all of the other resources available to you in your body, mind, and spirit to create a vibrant and meaningful life—a life worth living.

There is only one road to immortality and one thing of permanence, and that is love. If you live the circle of life, you will constantly rebirth yourself and, when you leave your body, your consciousness will educate those generations that follow with the gift of your love, spirit, and wisdom. This book can be your guide on that journey.

Bernie S. Siegel, M.D.

Introduction

There are two central issues that confront us as we explore the human potential to live long and healthy lives. The first is the reduction or compression of chronic illnesses, such as diabetes and heart disease. Medical science can already do this to some degree. In order to have the physical capacity and vitality to enjoy our golden years, we must take care of ourselves throughout our life span. In this book, you will discover just how to do this. With this knowledge, you will be primed to separate what's evidence-based from what's just sensational sales gimmickry.

There's a second, more complex issue in the whole longevity field, and that is the hotly debated scientific question of how long the human life span really can be. The longest-living human on record was a French woman, Jeanne Calment, who died in 1997 at the ripe old age of 122. Centenarians (people who have made it to 100) are one of the fastest-growing age groups in the United States. Some scientists predict that with new gene therapies and other scientific wizardry, we may even live to be 150 or older. The ongoing question will be whether in the expansion of years lived we are equally able to maintain the physical health of our organs and muscles so that those extra years are valuable to us and our loved ones. Given how much science and technology have exploded in only the past 50 years, we only hope to live long enough to witness some of the phenomenal longevity miracles we are certain are yet to be discovered.

There is no one secret to longevity. Rather, living a long and healthy life is the result of a happy marriage of many ingredients. In this book, you'll discover what those ingredients are and how to incorporate them into your own life for maximum life span and health span.

We wish you joy and vibrant good health on this amazing journey we call life.

How This Book Is Organized

This book is organized into four easy-to-follow parts. Each part covers an important component of the longevity lifestyle. Interested in one particular topic? Leaf through the pages and discover just what you need to know.

Part 1, "Secrets to Aging Well," provides an introduction to longevity and also looks at longevity from the perspective of your heredity and your age group. Part 1 also outlines all the screening tests currently recommended to help prevent illness and prolong life.

Part 2, "The Longevity Lifestyle," includes essential information about the longevity lifestyle—your nutrition, your physical fitness, and your weight, along with other vital components such as sleep and the importance of human touch and connection.

Part 3, "Longevity and Health: Knowledge Is Power," explores some specifics about how to keep your inner organs in tip-top shape, including your heart, your brain, and your musculoskeletal system. You'll also learn how to help prevent diabetes and cancer. Then we'll explore the impact of hormones as well as great skin care on your well-being and your longevity.

Part 4, "Passion for Life: The Ultimate Longevity Booster," reveals the power and impact of your mind and your spirit on your physical well-being and your long life. You'll explore what you're passionate about in this life, along with ways to create the life you were meant to live, so that every day of your life is imbued with purpose and satisfaction.

Extras

This book includes four different types of sidebars to enhance your understanding of longevity. Look for these boxes:

Doctors' Orders _____

Unsure if a specific practice, product, or procedure is safe? Check these boxes for cautions and concerns.

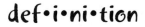

def•i•ni•tion _____

Medicalese can be confusing! Here you'll find definitions and explanations of medical terms that may be unfamiliar to you.

Longevity Facts _____

Look here for facts and instructive trivia about longevity.

Words to the Wise

You'll find helpful insights and other information in these boxes.

Acknowledgments

From Dr. Kay:

I would like to acknowledge my two sons, Neil and Ryan, who have taught me patience, compassion, selfless love, and surrender—and made me a much better physician than I would have otherwise been. My husband, Rob, for wearing the hats of househusband extraordinaire and phenomenal parent, while I have been busy on this book. My sister, Ann, and my mother, for teaching me the power of the soft arms of unconditional love. My father, for his philosophical and spiritual wisdom guiding me whenever needed.

I would like to thank my work angels—Ken Watson, for his steadfast encouragement and support in making it possible for me to write this book despite my job as a physician; my medical assistant, Armando, for caring for my patients when I was not there; and Dr. David Norene, for seeing and believing in me from the very beginning.

My in-laws and my friends, who have been my biggest fans; and my patients, in whose presence I have learned the true meaning of healing and who have taught me the true secrets to longevity.

And finally, and most importantly—my career partner and the yin to my yang—Max, without whom my career in complementary medicine and this book would have never taken place and with whom it has been a magical and exhilarating journey.

From Dr. Max:

I would like to acknowledge first and foremost my family—my wonderful husband, Don, who has encouraged and supported me through this entire book-writing process; my three amazing children, Davey, Doug, and Julia, who have been my greatest teachers and who have taught me love, compassion, and wisdom; and all the rest of my family, including my mom, who is one of my biggest heroes.

To my incredible friends who have encouraged me every step of the way, especially Elizabeth Bell; to David Norene, who recognized my dream and encouraged me to start; to my office staff who supported me throughout this process, helping me to take care of my patients as I worked to nurture this book along—they are my team extraordinaire; to my amazing colleague of over 15 years, Dr. Joi Barrett, who has always modeled for me what it means to be a phenomenal primary care physician; and to my patients, who have taught me how to be a physician and who always bring me the healing that I need in my own life.

And finally, my friend and colleague with whom I am privileged to work—Kay Judge, who calls forth greatness, grace, and possibility, not only in me but in everyone who is honored to know her; none of this amazing journey would have happened without her.

We would also like to acknowledge our colleagues who gave of their time generously to review our material and provide feedback to us:

Sallie Adams, M.D., FACE
Paul Akins, M.D.
Elizabeth Bell, R.N., DNS
Dorothy Breininger
Rari Coss, R.N.
Fran Fisher, R.N., Ph.D.

Ann Haas, M.D.

Sue Hazeghazam, R.D.

Julie Hersch, M.D.

Thomas Hopkins, M.D.

Risa MacDonald, PT, DPT

Ginger McMullen, M.D., FACE

Lydia Mendoza, LCSW

James Nishio, M.D.

Debbie Oudiz, Ph.D.

JaNahn Scalapino, M.D.

Robert Schott, M.D.

Dennis Warren, J.D.

Terri Wolf, R.N.

Lydia Wytrzes, M.D.

We also want to recognize the *Sacramento Bee* and McClatchy newspapers, through which we have had the opportunity to write a column on Integrative Medicine since October of 2005; Kevin McKenna, our editor at the *Bee*, was instrumental in creating this opportunity for us.

We wish to thank all of our editors at Alpha Books, including Lynn Northrup, development editor; Kayla Dugger, production editor; and Cate Schwenk, copy editor; they were masterful at reviewing our material with precision and making the final book shine. We would also like to thank Paul Dinas, senior acquisitions editor, for nurturing this project from the start and guiding us across the finish line!

And last but not least at all, we would like to acknowledge our fabulous book editor, Karen Brees, Ph.D., our master coach, cheerleader, and writing angel, who made us believe in this book and in ourselves every step of the way—what a privilege it's been!

Trademarks

Part 1

Secrets to Aging Well

What's the secret to maintaining a thriving life span and health span? It's no secret at all! Growing older doesn't have to mean falling apart. We all want to live well and live long. With the average life span of Americans hovering at 77 years, it's important to see what factors are involved in getting to that point and also moving beyond it. In this first part, we take a look at people and populations who have achieved longevity. We also explore your personal risk for illness and what types of medical screening tests can make a difference in your health and longevity.

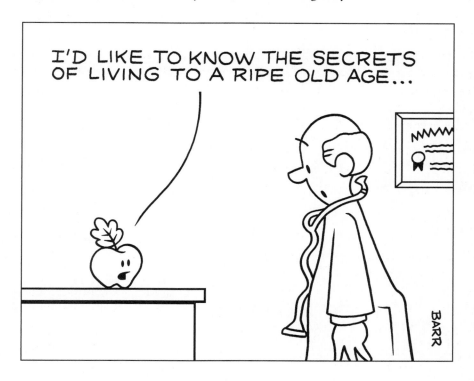

Chapter 1

Seeking a Great Health Span

In This Chapter

- Long life and great health
- Getting with the program: attitude is everything
- Getting past your genes
- The role of calorie restriction
- Confident and energized: body, mind, and spirit

What do we really want as we get older? Most of us are seeking not only a long life span, but vibrantly good health as well. We want to sustain our energy and vitality as we enter the next phase of our lives—our mature years. New research suggests that most of us can do just that, as long as we begin the process of taking care of ourselves now and stay active and involved in life. In this chapter, we'll start to explore what that means.

Many people are now living well past 90, and many of them are healthy and functioning well. The age-old myth of people falling apart once they hit their mid to later years is just that—a myth. When you start to look at the number of people who do live well and thrive into their later years, you'll see that it's possible for you, too. The *American Journal of Clinical Nutrition* reports that today about 1 in 10,000 people in the United States is 100 years old or older, and it is estimated that in the industrialized world that number will soon increase to 1 in 5,000. In this book, you will discover the tools you need to create the great health and well-being that will allow you to thrive into your 90s and beyond.

To 150 Years and Beyond!

At the turn of the last century, the average life expectancy in the United States was around 47. This was due in part to the high rate of child mortality and also to high mortality rates for women during childbirth. Medical technology, including high-tech surgical procedures, as well as improved sanitation, plentiful food supply, vaccinations, antibiotics, and the like, have contributed to prolonging life. Today, scientists predict that most of us will live well into our 80s; in fact, many predict that given the right environment, the human body is capable of living to 150 or longer.

Concerns

Alongside this, however, is the increasing rise of obesity, particularly in the United States, with its attendant risks of premature disability and death from cardiovascular disease, stroke, dementia, diabetes, and arthritis. Humans are capable of living far longer than we've ever imagined, but if that's our goal, then it's essential that we take care of the machinery that is our body so it's equipped to run smoothly for years to come.

Experts worry that if the current trend of obesity and sedentary lifestyle continues in the United States, people who are now middle-aged and younger will be the first ones in our history to actually have a *shorter* life span than their parents.

Longevity Facts

Jeanne Louise Calment has the oldest confirmed life span of any human being. A French woman from the town of Arles in southern France, she died in 1997 at the age of 122. She was still riding a bicycle until the age of 100 and lived on her own until she was about 110. She enjoyed good food and wine and also smoked cigarettes until the age of 119, when she reportedly quit only because she could no longer see well enough to light them! She attributed her own longevity to lots of laughter and a diet rich in olive oil (which she also used daily on her skin to keep it youthful-looking). She reportedly once said that she never wore mascara because she laughed until she cried too often.

Senescence

It wasn't that long ago scientists held pretty pessimistic views on aging. Senescence, or the biological changes associated with an aging body, as well as degenerative diseases, were felt to be almost inevitable; i.e., if you were lucky enough to make it into your later years, chances are you would be stuck with those chronic problems such as heart disease that we assumed came along with age. We know now, however, that while changes do take place in the body, they are not necessarily tied to inevitable deterioration and failure, as long as we commit to remaining healthy and vital for the long haul.

Why is longevity such a popular topic? It's probably because adults over the age of 65 are the fastest-growing segment of the population in the United States. The National Institute on Aging estimates that by the middle of the current century, there will be close to half a million people in the United States who will be centenarians, or over 100 years old.

Older folks today are healthier, wealthier, more educated, and more productive than older folks in previous times. Seniors are remaining active in society, and they have tremendous political clout; they are determined to have a voice in their own future. They are challenging *ageism*—the stereotypical view that Westerners tend to hold about older folks and their limited ability to contribute to society.

Longevity Facts

It is sometimes difficult to separate changes that inevitably occur with senescence from changes that are the result of poor lifestyle choices. What we previously thought was inevitable and irreversible, such as heart disease, is not only preventable, but also treatable with changes in lifestyle. Your hair may turn gray, but your heart can probably pump for a century, if you're kind to it.

Conceptualizing Age

We can think of age in several ways; two of the most common are chronological age and biological age. *Chronological age* refers to the number of years a person has actually lived. *Biological age*, on the other hand, is an estimate of age based on one's health parameters, using biomarkers such as blood pressure, muscle strength, and blood sugar level.

Dr. Michael Roizen, a highly respected physician and author of several works on the topic of aging, has popularized the concept of biological age. He refers to it as one's RealAge, which may be older or younger than your chronological age, depending on how well you've taken care of that body of yours. For example, if you smoke, you are felt to be biologically about 8 years older than your actual age because of the harm tobacco does; on the other hand, if you exercise regularly, burning up at least 3,500 calories per week, your RealAge is felt to be 3.4 years younger than your calendar age.

Normal aging, or usual aging, is the physical decline associated with the degenerative diseases so common in Western cultures, including heart disease, diabetes, dementia, tooth decay, and arthritis.

Successful aging refers to aging that is unaccompanied by chronic disease and disability. Successful aging is commonly seen in cultures where people live a traditional lifestyle with plenty of vigorous physical activity throughout their lives, ongoing engagement with meaningful work, community involvement, and nonprocessed diets.

Uncovering Longevity's Secrets

Scientists are starting to question the inevitability of physical decline. Perhaps we only appear to fall apart as we age because that's what so many of us have our focus on. How often have you heard people say, "I turned 50 and I started falling apart!" Perhaps no one has bothered to turn the lens on those folks who are aging with vim and vigor—those people who age beautifully and maintain their *health span* as well as their life span. Turns out there are plenty of people who are doing just that—and data about what those folks have in common is piling up.

def•i•ni•tion

> Your **health span** is the percentage of your life span that is spent in good health, where you have the energy and the vitality to pursue the activities that are important to you.

The MacArthur Foundation Study

The John D. and Catherine T. MacArthur Foundation is a private institution that makes grants to individuals and groups devoted to research and projects that create lasting improvement in the human condition, both in the United States and abroad.

In 1984, the MacArthur Foundation sponsored a group of scientists who proposed to study older people (as well as some older animals) over a period of years to determine which habits and genetic traits contributed the most to healthy aging. The researchers gathered knowledge about aging from many approaches—looking not only at bio-medical-genetic influences on aging, but also on the impact of physical activity, intellectual pursuits, social interactions, and the like, to generate a new concept about what it means to age successfully. What they found turned a lot of common assumptions on their ear. They published their book titled *Successful Aging* in 1998 (see Appendix B).

The MacArthur Foundation Study challenged many myths of aging, including the expectation that old age was inevitably associated with illness and disability, or that healthy aging was only possible if you happened to inherit the right genes from your parents. These scientists showed that choices made throughout adulthood in both lifestyle and attitude had a dramatic impact on healthy aging. They also showed that we should accept responsibility for those choices, if we want to maximize the enjoyment of our older years. In other words, successful aging is not an accident; it is largely an outcome of our own self-care.

They defined successful aging as an active, intentional, effort-requiring process that people engaged in over a lifetime, encompassing three key components:

1. Reduction or, better yet, prevention of risk factors for disease, such as obesity, smoking, and inactivity.

2. Ongoing physical and mental engagement, including staying physically active and engaging in intellectual pursuits that stimulate the brain.

3. Ongoing engagement in activities that bring meaning and purpose to one's life, including work activities, family time, social activities and organizations, as well as volunteerism.

The MacArthur study challenged and disproved several pervasive myths about aging, including the following:

- ◆ *Myth:* Physical and mental decline are inevitable as we age. *Fact:* Physical and mental decline have been shown to be reversible, given the appropriate training.

- ◆ *Myth:* Once disability has set in, it is irreversible. *Fact:* Chronic diseases are reversible with changes in lifestyle and attitude.

◆ *Myth:* Your genes are the main determinants of how you'll age. *Fact:* Only about 30 percent of physical aging and 50 percent of cognitive decline were shown to be due to one's genes. Furthermore, the influence of your genes becomes less important with every year you age, but your lifestyle becomes more important.

Lessons from Okinawa

The people of Okinawa—a group of islands located at the southern tip of Japan—boast the greatest longevity on the planet today. Living an average of over 81 years, their old age is generally spent in vigorous good health. What is their secret? Three physicians, including an Okinawan native, studied the people of this island nation as part of the Okinawa Centenarian Study and published their findings in their book titled *The Okinawa Program* (see Appendix B).

These researchers found that Okinawans eat a healthy diet high in plant foods—including seaweed, turmeric, goya, and tofu. The people in Okinawa living a traditional lifestyle remain active throughout their lives; they don't retire in the sense that Americans tend to retire. Community involvement is important to the islanders, and elders are considered a vital and active part of their community.

Biomarkers of Health

In 1991, Dr. Irwin Rosenberg and Dr. William Evans at the USDA Human Nutrition Research Center on Aging at Tufts University published their book *Biomarkers: The 10 Keys to Prolonging Vitality* (Fireside, 1992). In their ground-breaking work, they showed that aging could be slowed, stopped, or even reversed when people adhered to certain lifestyle principles. They identified a number of *biomarkers* they felt were most predictive of one's vitality and longevity. Most of these markers were affected by the level of physical activity in one's life. They included the following:

def•i•ni•tion

A **biomarker** is a physical characteristic or trait that is indicative of one's biological age or risk of illness.

◆ Lean body muscle mass—The sum weight of all muscle tissues in the body. This is determined by how much you use your muscles, as well as by the amount of androgenic (male) hormones circulating in your tissues. These hormones tend to drop off in both men and women as we age, so exercise becomes even more important as we get older.

- Physical strength—The ability of your muscles to lift or move weight. Without regular use, your muscles quickly atrophy or shrink and become weak.

- Basal metabolic rate (BMR)—The number of calories burned by your muscles, organs, and other tissues while you are at rest. If your muscle mass drops, so does your BMR.

- Body fat percentage—The percentage of your body tissue that is fat; this tends to rise with age, as your muscle mass decreases.

- Aerobic capacity—The body's ability to take up and use oxygen; the greater your muscle mass and the more fit you are, the more oxygen you use and the greater your aerobic capacity is.

- Blood pressure—The pressure generated in your arteries as your heart contracts and relaxes. In Western cultures, blood pressure tends to rise with age, and this increases the risk of cardiovascular disease.

- Insulin sensitivity—The ability of your tissues to respond to insulin so that they can take up and use glucose (sugar) in your blood. Obesity reduces insulin sensitivity, leading to elevated blood sugar.

- Total cholesterol/HDL cholesterol ratio—HDL is the protective cholesterol in the body and reduces your risk of heart disease. It tends to drop as you age and also if you develop diabetes. An ideal total cholesterol to HDL ratio is less than 4.

- Bone density—A measure of the strength of your bones. Bone density tends to drop as you get older, especially if you are sedentary and not getting enough nutrients, such as vitamin D and calcium. Bed rest also leads to loss of bone density.

What was the underlying theme in all of these biomarkers? You guessed it—exercise. Other than quitting smoking, these researchers showed that the single best thing people could do to increase vitality, health, and longevity at any age was to exercise (we'll give you lots of information about healthy exercise in Chapter 5).

Between the ages of 20 and 70, we lose about 30 percent of our muscle cells; this loss happens gradually—equaling almost 7 pounds of lean body muscle mass every 10 years. The effect is cumulative. We hit 70 and we wonder why it seems hard to get out of a chair or why it seems easy to fall. However, daily aerobic exercise, combined with stretching and weight training, was shown to help people regain muscle mass that had been lost even by years of disuse. Patients in their studies increased the *size* of their muscle mass by up to 12 percent and also doubled and at times tripled their strength. These changes were the foundation of all of the other biomarkers, as healthy muscle mass and strength drives all of the others.

Here's the other important point: with a program of regular exercise and strength training, these researchers showed that people of any age (including those in their late 90s) can increase their aerobic and strength capacity and reduce their biological age by as much as 20 years.

Optimism and Longevity

Many studies have shown that optimism increases longevity, and lest you worry because you consider yourself a pessimist, rest assured that optimism can be a learned trait. Here is a smattering of those studies:

◆ In the 1960s, the Mayo Clinic in Rochester, Minnesota, surveyed over 800 incoming patients who were self-referred for medical care. These patients completed a series of questionnaires, including a screening for the trait of optimism. When this group was reevaluated in 2000, the optimists were found to have significantly greater longevity than the pessimists.

◆ In the 1930s, the The Nun Study was begun. This ingenious investigation looked at the impact of positive emotion and optimism on the longevity of a group of Roman Catholic nuns. The researchers found that nuns who scored high on tests of optimism were not only healthier than their grouchier comrades, they also lived longer.

◆ A study of over 2,200 older Mexican Americans living in the southwest United States found that those who scored the highest on tests for positive emotion not only looked younger but also had half the death and disability rate of their pessimistic counterparts. The study was reported in the May 2000 issue of the *Journal of the American Geriatric Society.*

◆ In the late 1930s, Harvard University initiated what is now called The Harvard Study of Adult Development, the world's longest-running study of what it takes to age successfully. It started out with a cohort of young men who were sophomores at Harvard College and then incorporated two other groups: a group of teenagers from inner-city Boston, as well as a cohort of young women from California. The participants have been studied and interviewed as often as every two years since the onset; most of them are now over 80. Dr. George Vaillant, the current director of the study, has identified a number of factors common to those in the study who have aged well, aged successfully, and enjoyed long life. These include:

- Gratitude, forgiveness, altruism, love, empathy, friendship, joy, and a sense of grace

- The capacity to plan and hope for the future

- Curiosity, initiative, creativity, playfulness, and a sense of humor

- Level of education

- Ongoing development of new friendships and intimate connections, especially as older friends pass away

- A satisfying marriage

- Caring about people

- Reframing life's difficult moments as opportunities for growth

- Acceptance of the changes that come with age

Interestingly, a good marriage in midlife predicted successful aging at the age of 80, but a low blood cholesterol level did not offer the same protection. Alcohol abuse predicted poor aging, mainly because it disrupted relationships. Regular exercise, maintenance of a healthy weight, and avoidance of tobacco were also important, but not as much as the other factors listed above.

Human Connection and Longevity

Numerous studies have shown that strong social connections enhance health and longevity, even if personal health habits are not ideal. One of the most well known of these studies is the Roseto, Pennsylvania Study. Roseto is a small town in eastern Pennsylvania whose inhabitants in the 1950s were found to have a much lower rate of heart attacks and death from heart disease compared to the rest of the country, despite the fact that many of its inhabitants smoked and had high-fat diets and diabetes. Why the difference?

Roseto was settled in the late 1800s by a group of immigrants from a town in southern Italy. At the onset of the study, Roseto still consisted largely of these closely knit Italian families. In the 1960s and 1970s however, as young family members left Roseto and the community became fragmented, the rate of heart disease rose, and the mortality rates became the same as those of neighboring communities.

In the 1970s through the 1990s, numerous other studies done in communities around the world found the same thing: people with strong social ties and strong community involvement had up to an 80 percent reduction in all-cause mortality compared to those who were socially isolated. Social connection again appeared to be a more powerful predictor of longevity than healthy lifestyle habits. And social involvement *plus* healthy habits was the most powerful recipe for longevity. You'll read more about the association of human connection and longevity in Chapter 9.

Longevity and Your Belief System

Is aging and longevity affected by our beliefs and attitudes, especially when these beliefs are shared and reinforced by the culture in which we reside? The answer is probably yes, though data on this is just emerging.

In 1979, Dr. Ellen Langer, a renowned psychologist at Harvard, did an ingenious experiment to examine the impact of awareness and attention on the process of aging. Her theory was that biological aging was influenced by whether or not people *experienced* themselves as old. She and her colleagues recruited a group of healthy men, all age 75 or older, to attend a week-long retreat at a local resort. The men were told they were being evaluated for their physical and mental health. They were also told not to bring any written or printed materials with them that were dated after 1959.

When the men arrived at the retreat center, they found it had been set up as if the year was 1959. The books, newspapers, furnishings, music, and so forth were all from 1959. The participants were then asked to spend the week behaving as if it really was 1959; this meant speaking only about events from 1959 in the present tense, as well as imagining themselves, their families, and their friends to be 20 years younger. In fact, they all had ID badges with photos that had been taken in 1959 to help them relate to one another as younger men. In addition to this group of men, there was a control group of men at the retreat who were not involved in this 1959 scheme. The researchers made a number of physical and cognitive measurements of the men at the beginning and then again at the end of the week.

What they found was nothing short of amazing; there were improvements in parameters of aging that prior to this study were felt to be irreversible. Compared to the 1979 men, the 1959 group showed an improvement in physical and mental function—including memory, physical independence, physical activity, and agility. Their joints were more flexible; they were less stiff; they were physically stronger; and their hearing, vision, and posture were all improved. Their finger length was also increased (finger length tends to go down with age). Over 50 percent of the 1959 group also showed an increase on IQ test scores, while 25 percent of those in the control group actually had a reduction in their IQ scores. Finally, an independent group of people evaluated photos of the men taken at the beginning and again at the end of the week and reported that the men looked younger by about three years at the end of the experiment.

Dr. Langer wrote about this study in her book *Mindfulness* (Da Capo Press, 1989). While it was difficult to be certain which specific interventions had led to the positive changes in these men, she estimated that the results were probably due to several factors, including the fact that the men were treated as if they really were 20 years younger, they were expected to behave as if they were younger, and they were also felt to be capable of carrying out complex tasks that might otherwise only be expected of younger men.

What does this mean for us? It certainly challenges the notion that aging is an inevitable downhill slide. It behooves all of us to pay attention to our attitudes about aging, not only for ourselves, but for those around us as well.

Is There an Anti-Aging Gene?

Researchers have long looked for an anti-aging gene, something that would predict who is destined to live a long and healthy life. For example, some scientists have noted that those who are blessed with genetically healthy lipoproteins, those compounds that carry cholesterol and other fats in our blood, seem more likely to make it to 100.

Studies conducted using worms have shown that the alteration of a gene called daf-2 will extend life. This gene, which has also been found in mice and fruit flies, seems to be the master controller of metabolism in these creatures. In yeast, a gene called sir-2 seems to get turned on by calorie restriction, and calorie restriction, as we discuss in the following section, is associated with longevity in animals.

Researchers are actively looking for genes that might be similarly powerful in humans. The hormone *insulin* is probably part of this human gene system, because insulin and several other growth factors are the main players in human energy metabolism. Excess insulin, which is seen in overweight or obese patients with pre- and adult-onset diabetes, is associated with a shortened life span in humans.

def•i•ni•tion

Insulin is a hormone made by the pancreas. It is considered one of the master regulators of metabolism in the body and is primarily responsible for the metabolism of glucose. If insulin becomes deficient or if it stops working efficiently, then diabetes develops.

Another newly discovered cellular process that seems to affect aging, as well as the risk of diseases such as cancer, is called autophagy. Autophagy is the ability of a cell to literally devour and remove parts of itself that are old and unhealthy—parts that if left untouched could harm the cell. The first autophagy gene identified in humans was called beclin-1. Studies in both animals and humans have shown that if this gene is defective or missing, the risk of cancer is increased, including cancers of the breast, ovary, and prostate. Inactivation of this gene in animals can also reduce life span. Stay tuned for more data in the near future, as researchers look for ways to activate this gene to reduce disease and increase longevity.

This new gene research is exciting, and one day aging may be vastly different from the way we now experience it. In the meantime, however, the best way to assure yourself of a long life span and health span is to cultivate optimism and altruism, maintain your social connectivity, and embrace a healthy lifestyle, including the avoidance of obesity.

Eat Less, Live Longer

Calorie restriction is an idea that goes back to the 1930s, when it was noticed that laboratory rodents lived almost twice as long as normal and maintained their youthful appearance if their food intake was restricted while their nutrient intake was maintained. They were also less likely to suffer from age-related diseases; in other words, they aged with gusto.

Calorie Restriction (CR)

When following Calorie Restriction with Optimal Nutrition (CRON), subjects are fed far fewer calories than usual, but nutrient needs are met. The Calorie Restriction Society was formed in 1994 by devotees of this practice; its members practice calorie restriction (CR) as a means of prolonging life *and* maintaining good health—an essential combination if you want to enjoy those additional years!

Most studies of calorie restriction have been done in lab animals, including rodents and worms; so far, reduced chronic disease (including cancer and Alzheimer's disease) and increased life spans have been observed in just about every living organism tested. Studies in humans are much fewer in number, however. In humans, calorie restriction generally leads to weight loss and reduced blood pressure, blood glucose, and lipids; these are great benefits in and of themselves, leading to a reduced risk of developing diabetes, hypertension, and heart disease, or a reduced severity of disease for those already diagnosed with these conditions.

Doctors' Orders _____

Are there risks to CR? If adequate nutrition is not maintained and weight loss is too severe, this approach becomes more harmful than good and can increase one's risk of malnutrition, muscle wasting, and osteoporosis. In addition, CR seems to make ALS (Lou Gehrig's disease) worse and is not recommended for children and teens. We recommend that you talk with your doctor before embarking on a CR lifestyle.

However, there seems to be something more going on here than just the benefits of weight loss. There are a number of theories as to why CRON not only reduces chronic disease and extends the life span, but also delays aging and extends the health span. These theories propose a number of mechanisms:

◆ Reduction of *free radicals* in the body

◆ Activation of longevity enzymes or genes

◆ Reduction of DNA instability

◆ Lowered metabolism

◆ Increased levels of growth hormone

◆ Reduced harmful effects of excess glucose and insulin in the bloodstream

def•i•ni•tion _____

Free radicals, molecules with unstable unpaired electrons, are capable of damaging other molecules or cells. Free radicals are generated by normal cellular metabolism and also by environmental substances, such as cigarette smoke and radiation. Antioxidants are nutrients or chemicals such as vitamin C that quench or neutralize these electrons and prevent them from causing damage.

Is there an overlying reason for this increase in longevity with calorie restriction? In nature, when food shortages occur, all organisms seem to slow down metabolically to conserve precious resources. And because nature is committed to the perpetuation of its species and adequate food is necessary for reproduction, animals deprived of calories will delay their reproduction until adequate nutrition is available. This delay also ends up prolonging the total life span of those animals.

Resveratrol

Researchers are also studying chemicals that seem to stimulate the beneficial effects of CR, even if the organism does not reduce caloric intake (oh, happy day!). These include resveratrol, a plant nutrient found in red wine and the skin of red grapes.

Resveratrol has anti-inflammatory actions, protects many tissues in the body (including the heart), and also seems to protect against cancer. Perhaps this is why some people who enjoy red wine in moderation seem less likely to suffer from heart disease. Resveratrol is produced by grapes and other plants when they are grown in stressful environments, such as when growing conditions and nutrient availability are poor, similar to calorie restriction. In addition, there are other substances that work in similar ways to resveratrol, including alpha-lipoic acid, as well as Metformin (a.k.a. Glucophage), a drug used to treat type 2 diabetes.

Another approach being studied to promote longevity is intermittent calorie restriction (i.e., restricting calories every other day). For those of you who can't bear the thought of semistarvation every day, this may produce the same benefit.

We'll go into more detail about an anti-inflammatory diet in Chapter 4.

Body, Mind, and Spirit

So how do we put this all together? How do we sum up all of what's known so far about healthy aging? New data will continue to emerge on this topic every year, and hopefully we will continue to challenge our, at times, limited beliefs about what is possible for human beings.

First and foremost, for the vast majority, taking care of your body is paramount to living well and living long. The biggest bang for your buck probably comes from remaining physically vigorous throughout your life, including getting plenty of aerobic exercise, maintaining your muscle mass, and keeping those muscles stretched.

Also important is the consumption of as healthy a diet as possible, with loads of produce, whole grains, healthy protein, and limited animal fat. As you get older, you need fewer calories to maintain your weight every year, so with the reduced need for calories, it's even more important that what you do eat is packed with nutrients and not wasted junk calories. Finally, limiting your body's exposure to toxins is also important; this includes tobacco, excess alcohol, recreational drugs, and environmental chemicals and toxins, where possible.

Equally important is your mental health. Some of us seem to have been born lucky optimists, but many of us dip into the morass of pessimistic thinking a little more often than is good for our mental well-being. The good news is that with practice and persistence, you can learn to change this and create a more optimistic outlook on your life. Just as your muscles will quickly wither if you go to bed and become a slug, so, too, will your mind lapse back into negative thinking if you don't exercise your power of practice and choice in this matter.

Longevity Facts

A healthy mental outlook, including practiced optimism and the expectation of healthy aging, seems to increase longevity.

Finally, there's the spiritual realm. This includes the power of intimacy and connection with other human beings (especially family), generating a sense of meaning and purpose in our lives, living our lives with intention, having a positive expectation for the future, and practicing gratitude and forgiveness. These have all been shown to have a huge impact on happiness, well-being, *and* longevity.

Will we live forever? Not in the current human paradigm in which we dwell. But can we live our lives in such a way that dramatically increases our life span as well as our health span? That ensures we will not just *survive* our later years, but *thrive* throughout most of our lives? That minimizes disability and expands our capacity for full participation in life? The answer is an unequivocal yes; the power and the possibility for a long and fulfilling life are in your hands.

The Least You Need to Know

- ◆ Many people are living and thriving now into their 90s and beyond.
- ◆ Growing old with great health means cultivating great health habits *now*—regular exercise, healthy diet, avoiding toxins, staying involved in your community, and generating optimism.
- ◆ Your attitudes and expectations about aging probably have a large impact on how you will ultimately fare.
- ◆ Calorie restriction, or at the very l____ a lean and healthy weight, may increase your longevity.
- ◆ In the future, genetic therapie____ ____ronic disease and live longer and healthier live____

Understanding Your Longevity Group

In This Chapter

- Risk factors by age group
- Considerations for men and women
- Your family tree
- The role ethnicity plays
- Genetics and longevity

Different populations of people have different life spans. This may not be fair, but it's fact. For example, the average American woman lives 5.3 years longer than the average American man. In this chapter, we'll examine why this is and take a look at the roles gender, ethnicity, age, and genetics play in your health span and your life span.

Longevity and Your Age Group

Each age group has certain risk factors that can negatively impact longevity. Understanding those risk factors can help you make positive lifestyle changes to increase your longevity. Here's a breakdown by age on the longevity challenges you are likely to encounter.

Ages 1–44

According to the Centers for Disease Control (CDC), the leading cause of death for this age group is unintentional injury. Unintentional injuries (accidents), homicide, and suicide are responsible for 75 percent of deaths for those aged 15 to 19, 72 percent of deaths for those aged 20 to 24, and 54 percent of deaths for those aged 25 to 34 years.

> **Words to the Wise**
>
> If you know your personal health risks, you can develop strategies to improve your health and increase your longevity. A great deal is within your control!

Longevity secrets for this age group: Avoid accidents! Treat depression and seek help if you are in a violent relationship or if you're experiencing suicidal thoughts. This is the time to begin leading a lifestyle you want to maintain for the rest of your life. Avoid excessive sun exposure. Exercise regularly. Learn to deal with stress. Don't smoke and avoid secondhand smoke.

Ages 45–54

Cancer, heart disease, and accidents are the top three killers in this age group.

Longevity secrets for this age group: Start your cancer screenings. Be aware of your family history and start early screenings, including cholesterol and blood sugar, if you are at risk. Drive carefully. Wear a helmet if you ride a bike. Stop smoking if you are a smoker. Get to your ideal weight. Learn to live the life you have always wanted and to manage stress effectively.

Age 55–64

Cancer and heart disease remain the top two killers here, and lung diseases and diabetes move up to numbers three and four.

Longevity secrets for this age group: Don't smoke—try to quit, if you are smoking. Make sure you are getting tested for your cholesterol, blood pressure, and blood sugars to prevent or treat any developing problems. Maintain your goal weight. Find love, passion, and meaning in your life. This is the time of transitioning—of empty nests and ending careers. Start to find out what life is all about for you. This will give you the energy and motivation to live a long, healthy life.

Ages 65–74

Cancer, heart disease, and lung disease are numbers one, two, and three in causes of mortality here. Stroke moves up to number four.

Longevity secrets for this age group: Stay active and stay healthy. Continue regular screenings and make sure you are seeing your physician regularly. Do not ignore warning signs that could be indicators of a stroke or heart attack. Seek counseling or help if you are depressed or socially isolated. Volunteer or start a hobby if you are retired. Give and get love—if you don't have close social relationships, then pets can provide comfort, love, and a chance to exercise!

Ages 75–84

Heart disease moves up to number one. Cancer, stroke, lung disease, and diabetes round out numbers two through five as causes of mortality in this sector.

Longevity secrets for this age group: Maintain that healthy heart. Continue yearly physicals. Use it or lose it! Stay healthy, active, and socially connected. Continue to find ways to make life's journey meaningful. Forgive and move forward. Be graceful and positive about your health.

Ages 85 and Over

Heart disease, cancer, stroke, Alzheimer's, and influenza and pneumonia are the top killers in this age group.

Longevity secrets for this age group: You are on your way to the century mark! Keep up your great lifestyle and keep up good routine maintenance in your health. Keep up your strength and stability of gait. You may want to periodically streamline your medication list with your physician, discontinuing medications that may not be needed or may be causing adverse side effects. Stay socially connected and spiritually vibrant.

Your Gender

Despite recent increases in male life expectancy, women outlive men in all but the poorest countries. However, a lifestyle that is focused on reducing cardiovascular disease and decreasing cancer risk is guaranteed to improve your life span, regardless of your gender.

The source of greatest disadvantage for men under age 45 is behaviors attributable to gender. Men have an increased rate of accidental injuries compared to their female counterparts. Accidents, injuries, and suicides account for the majority of male mortality excess in this group and for more male than female deaths amongst all but the most elderly. Before the age of 60, risk-taking behavior claims more male lives than heart disease.

Cancer and heart disease are the two top causes of death for both men and women. Since the 1980s, however, men's mortality from cancer has exceeded women's mortality from the same disease. Diabetes and kidney disease occur with equal frequency in men and women.

Longevity Facts

In 2003, unintentional injuries were the third leading cause of death for males but the seventh for females. Suicide ranked eighth for males but was not ranked among the 10 leading causes for females. Alzheimer's disease ranked tenth for males but fifth for females. Because women tend to live longer than men, they may have more of a prevalence of Alzheimer's disease, which tends to appear later in life.

Men and Accidents

Accidents claim 90,000 lives a year—most of these victims are men, who are twice as likely to die from falls and more than three times as likely to die from accidental drowning. Men are also more likely to sustain head injuries. The increased risk of accidents is true for every age group of men, with the highest risk up to age 35.

Overall, men are three times more likely than women to die in car accidents, and men over 65 are twice as likely to be killed in car accidents than are females. Men over 75 are twice as likely to die as a result of an accident than their female counterparts.

The leading causes of all accidental deaths in adults are motor vehicle accidents, falls, poisonings, fires, and drowning.

Fall Precautions for Men and Women

Falls are the second leading cause of accidental death in the United States, with three quarters of them occurring in the older adult population.

Among the elderly, falls and hip fractures are the most common causes of accidental deaths. One third of older adults who fall and sustain a hip fracture and are hospitalized die within a year of the fall. Decrease your chances of falling and you will enhance your longevity. Here are some precautions you can take:

♦ Use a properly fitted cane, walker, or assistive device, if you have an unsteady gait.

♦ Have periodic eye exams or checkups, as decreased vision makes falls more likely.

♦ When possible, avoid medications causing dizziness—these can include blood pressure medications, narcotics, anxiety medications, and sleeping pills. Review your prescription medicines and over-the-counter medications with your physician to see if there are alternative medications that do not affect your balance and steadiness.

♦ Keep your muscles and joints well conditioned. There is a gradual decline in balance and speed of gait that occurs with age. These two are linked with activity level. Remaining physically active can help you avoid falls.

Here are some tips for fall-proofing your home:

♦ Wear good flat-heeled shoes with rubber soles for added traction.

♦ Avoid walking around in socks, stockings, or floppy, backless slippers at home.

♦ Avoid lifting anything over 20 pounds.

♦ Avoid activities that put compressive forces on your spine, such as opening a stuck window, as this may cause fractures of the spine.

♦ Place handrails where needed. Use night-lights.

♦ Keep a flashlight and a phone next to your bed.

♦ Avoid slippery floors or floors that get slippery when wet. Fix any uneven flooring that may cause falls.

♦ Eliminate the use of throw rugs, if possible. At the very least, avoid loose edges by taping the rug to the floor or using nonskid mats underneath the rug.

- Use shower bars and bath chairs in your bathroom to improve safety.

- Eliminate clutter on the floors and in pathways. This includes extension cords, stacks of papers, extra furniture with sharp edges, and boxes.

- For the outdoors, check for uneven sidewalks, terrain, or curbs requiring repair or highlighting. Keep the exterior of your home well lit; automatic lights are a plus.

Your Family History

Your health is the result of a combination of many factors—lifestyle, environment, habits, and genetics. Many diseases that threaten longevity have a genetic component to them. If there is a family tendency toward a particular illness, there is an increased likelihood that, at some point in your life, you may get that illness. But the important thing to realize about genetic tendencies is that much of the time they are not written in stone. Just because you have a family history or carry the genes for certain traits does not necessarily mean you will get that illness. Become knowledgeable about your family history and proactive in managing your health care! Knowing what you are predisposed to can help you screen for the illness and be on the alert should symptoms of that illness develop.

There are a few diseases that occur in our later years that are linked to family history, and you should be aware of them. They include heart attack, stroke, Alzheimer's disease, depression, alcoholism, diabetes, and osteoporosis. There are also many cancers that have a strong genetic tendency.

If you have a strong family history of a certain condition—if all your siblings and your parents have adult onset diabetes, for example—there is an increased likelihood that you will also develop this condition. Unfortunately, you can't change your genes. However, you *can* partner with your physician in reducing harmful health behaviors, such as smoking, inactivity, and poor eating habits.

If you have a family history of chronic disease, you may be able to prevent the disease just by making lifestyle changes. In the example of a family history of diabetes, reducing your weight may reduce your tendency to develop diabetes—even if you have a genetic tendency to get it.

It's also important to know that some diseases are not due to your genes, but rather to your lifestyle. And lifestyle and habits are learned behaviors that we pick up from our family. For example, if everyone in the family smoked, didn't exercise, and were overweight, there may be a strong family history of heart disease. Choosing not to smoke, exercising regularly, eating right, and watching your cholesterol may reverse your tendency to follow in your family's path of early heart disease.

Aggressive, appropriate, and early screening for early detection in people who have a family history of a chronic disease may pay great health dividends. Specific screening tests look for risk factors or early signs of disease. Finding disease early will certainly increase your odds of improving your health span and increasing your life span.

> **Words to the Wise**
>
> Genetics may load the gun, but environment pulls the trigger.
> —Pamela Peeke, M.D., M.P.H., *Fight Fat After Forty* (2000)

Conduct your own family history and inform your doctor of your findings at your yearly physical exam. For each family member you discover with a medical problem, write down the pertinent health history: health, weight, and lifestyle. Include habits such as smoking and any relevant environmental exposures to toxins. For example, your sister Mary had an early heart attack at age 55, weighed 200 pounds, and was an adult-onset diabetic. Keep this file with your medical records.

Here's a list of medical conditions that may have a family connection and should be noted in your family history:

- Cancer (include the age when the cancer occurred)
- Heart disease or stroke, especially at an early age (under 55 in men and under 65 for women)
- High blood pressure
- Stroke
- Alzheimer's disease
- Diabetes
- Asthma
- Mental illness, including bipolar disorder, schizophrenia, anxiety, or depression
- Alcoholism or drug abuse
- Autoimmune disease, such as lupus or rheumatoid arthritis
- Kidney disease
- Vision or hearing loss at a young age

When you are evaluating family history, it may be hard to distinguish important clues that may lead to an increased risk for you for that disease. Look for the following patterns in significant diseases in your family:

◆ Early disease; for example, prostate cancer at 80 may not be terribly significant, but a family history of prostate cancer at 50 may be. Diseases that occur at an earlier age than expected—about 10 or 20 years before their expected occurrence—are important in family history.

◆ Diseases that occur in multiple relatives, or in more than one close relative.

◆ Disease that does not usually affect a certain gender (e.g., breast cancer in a male).

◆ Certain combinations of diseases within a family (for example, breast and ovarian cancer, or heart disease and diabetes).

Having any of the above in your family history may provide important clues to diseases that may impact your longevity.

Your Ethnicity

The good news is that overall, as a nation, our longevity is improving. On the whole we are getting healthier and living longer, but this is not true across the racial divide. Certain ethnicities and racial groups continue to have more illness and higher death rates than others. Health education, finances, and access to health care are important factors.

Longevity Facts

Increased illness may, in small part, be due to genetic tendencies. For example, the Ashkenazi Jewish population (Jews of Eastern European descent) have a mutation in their genes that causes a 27-fold increased risk of breast cancer.

There may also be cultural differences in health behaviors, such as food, exercise, and approach to medical care. These issues may influence lifestyle behaviors and cause a shorter life span.

If you are a member of a minority ethnic group, it's important to note that there are substantial differences in longevity within certain ethnicities. Knowing your ethnic risk factors in advance can help you avoid these health pitfalls and improve your personal longevity.

Whereas individual ethnicities have some variation in how they fare with certain diseases, we still have to worry about cancer, heart disease, and stroke as the three major killers, regardless of our ethnicity. However, many of the health and lifestyle measures that improve longevity—and decrease the three major killers—will work in all racial groups to increase the life span within each group.

African American

According to the Centers for Disease Control, data shows that, over the last decades, the death rate from cancer is 25 percent higher in African Americans than for white Americans. Prostate cancer death rate is double that of whites and breast cancer death is also higher, even though mammogram screening rates are similar.

Forty-nine percent of African Americans die from direct complications of diabetes as opposed to 23 percent of Caucasians.

Death rates from HIV/AIDS are seven times that of whites, and the rates of homicide are six times that of whites.

Influenza vaccination coverage for adults 65 and older averages 52 percent in African Americans compared to 70 percent for the white population.

Hispanic

Hispanics are two times more likely to die of diabetes than are non-Hispanic whites.

Hispanics have an increased rate of contracting tuberculosis and also have a higher rate of hypertension and obesity than the general population.

Asian or Pacific Islander (API)

The good news is that Asian or Pacific Islanders (API) are very healthy as a population group. Certain groups have increased risks, however, for certain conditions. For example, cervical cancer occurs five times as often in the Vietnamese population than in the white population. Rates of tuberculosis and hepatitis are higher in the Asian population.

In comparing the three leading causes of death among the various ethnicities, for the Asian or Pacific Islander population, cancer was the leading cause of death, with heart disease second.

Heart disease and cancer were the first and second leading causes of death, respectively, for the white, black, and American Indian or Alaska Native populations. Stroke was the third leading cause of death for the white, black, and API populations.

The Role of Genetics

What do your *genetics* say about your longevity? Genetic testing holds great potential for helping increase our longevity. We are now learning that we can diagnose the genetic tendencies of certain individuals to develop certain diseases. In the years to come, scientists may be able to accurately predict much of your health risks by ana-lyzing your genetic structure.

def•i•ni•tion

> **Genetics** is the science of heredity and variation in human beings. It is based on the premise that molecules called DNA make up the genetic code of an individual and pat-terns in this genetic code determine various traits and disease states.

Genetic testing may be our proverbial crystal ball, gazing into our health future. We may find that we are predisposed to breast cancer, have a tendency to develop Alzheimer's, or be likely to develop diabetes. We may find we will respond better to certain medications than we do to others. We may find that we have a tendency toward addictive behaviors or depression. At this particular time, genetic testing in adults can be used to ...

- Discover if someone has a gene for a disease that might be passed on to his or her children.

- Test for certain genetic diseases before symptoms develop.

- Test high-risk groups, such as those with a family history of cancers, to see if a change in diagnosis and treatment plan is appropriate (for example, earlier and more frequent screenings, preventive medications, or other specific treatments).

- Confirm a diagnosis in a person who has symptoms of a particular disease.

Prediction, Not Diagnosis

Genetic testing does have some drawbacks that limit its universal use as a general screening tool for health problems. First, genetic tests are predictive. Predictive tests are those that do not give a yes/no answer. They can only tell what the *chances* are of developing a particular genetic condition. A genetic test only lets us know whether a specific genetic variant, or mutation, exists. However, it cannot predict whether the disease will actually develop.

There are many factors associated with developing a disease—especially those that are the most commonly associated with longevity, such as coronary artery disease, type 2 diabetes, obesity, and Alzheimer's disease. Just because the genes for these diseases exist does not mean that the diseases will develop. Lifestyle and environment also play a big role in determining whether the diseases occur.

Ethical and Legal Concerns

Genetic testing also leads to serious ethical and legal issues. One of these issues is patient privacy. There is a potential that the possibility of a future disease may lead to someone being declared ineligible for health insurance or life insurance coverage.

There are currently over 1,000 available genetic tests for specific diseases, including tests for the following:

- ◆ Huntington's disease (midlife onset; degenerative neurological disease)

- ◆ Polycystic kidney disease (cysts in the kidneys and other organs)

- ◆ Sickle cell disease (blood cell disorder)

- ◆ Tay-Sachs disease (neurological disease of early childhood)

- ◆ Thalassemias (reduced red blood cell levels)

def•i•ni•tion

Genetic tests (also called DNA-based tests) are laboratory tests for genetic disorders that an individual may have, and involve direct examination of the DNA molecule itself. The DNA sample can be obtained from any tissue, including blood.

If you decide to get tested, you may want to find out if your insurance covers the cost of testing. Many times the genetic tests run a few hundred dollars and are not covered by insurance. The National Human Genome Research Institute, the National Office of Public Health Genomics Centers for Disease Control and Prevention, and "Gene-tests" (a publication put out by the University of Washington) can give you more information on genetic testing.

If you have a strong family history of a genetically passed-on condition, knowing that you are at risk for it should motivate you to change your health management practices and possibly consider getting genetic testing. If, however, there is no benefit to testing, but rather the chance that it may lead to further worrying or potential hassles, you may want to defer genetic testing.

The Least You Need to Know

◆ Increase your longevity by focusing on the health risk factors for your age group.

◆ Know that gender plays a role in determining diseases you are likely to get.

◆ Falls lead to fractures and death. Learn what you need to do to fall-proof your surroundings.

◆ A family history of certain diseases can give us a clue to our risk factors for developing these diseases.

◆ Your ethnicity may be a risk factor for certain diseases.

◆ Genetic testing holds promise for early diagnosis and treatment of certain diseases.

Chapter 3

Keeping Healthy, Keeping Track

In This Chapter

- ◆ Essential facts on essential tests
- ◆ Controversial screenings
- ◆ United States Preventive Services Task Force recommendations for men and women
- ◆ Recovering quickly from surgery

Want to maximize your health span and your life span? Of course you do! Knowledge is the first step toward healthy living, and getting the recommended screenings for your age is the first line of defense. Don't be among the 50 percent of the population who neglect this aspect of health care. Be proactive and stay healthy. Familiarize yourself with the tests and screenings you need for your age and your gender.

Important Tests and Screenings

There are many tests and screenings available to you, but a few tests out there are guaranteed to help you live longer. Make sure you are getting these at the recommended age. Here's a look at these potential lifesavers.

Mammogram Screening

Mammography is a low-dose x-ray used to examine the breasts to aid in the diagnosis of breast diseases in women. Women who are over the age of 40 should have a screening mammogram with or without a clinical breast exam every one or two years. Patients with an increased risk of breast cancer include those with a family history of breast cancer in a mother or a sister, a previous biopsy revealing atypical hyperplasia, or a first childbirth after the age of 30. These patients are more likely to benefit from a screening mammogram than women who are at lower risk.

Longevity Facts

Clinical trials have shown there is a 30 percent reduction in death from breast cancer in women aged 50 to 69 who have an annual or biennial mammogram screening. Mammography plays a crucial role in early detection of breast cancers, because it can show changes in the breast up to two years before a patient or physician can feel these changes.

Make sure your mammograms are accurate. According to the American Cancer Society, the following is what you need to know to ensure you are getting good mammography screening:

- Do not wear deodorant, talcum powder, or lotion under your arms or on your breasts on the day of the exam. These can appear on the mammogram as calcium spots, which may be mistaken for abnormal findings.

- Describe any breast symptoms or problems to the technician performing the exam.

- If possible, obtain prior mammograms and make them available to the radiologist at the time of the current exam.

- Ask when your results will be available; do not assume the results are normal, if you do not hear from your doctor or the mammography facility.

The age at which mammograms should be discontinued is uncertain. Women older than 75 do have a higher risk of dying from breast cancer than do younger women, but they also have a higher risk of dying from other causes as well. If you are healthy and vital, you may want to continue mammography screening, regardless of your age.

Pap Smear

A pap smear takes a sample of cells from a woman's cervix to check for early changes suggestive of cervical cancer. Screening should start three years after onset of sexual activity or at age 21 (whichever comes first) and become part of your routine physical exam.

The U.S. Preventive Services Task Force found that screening was low yield in women after 65 who had had regular prior screenings. For older women who have had a history of normal pap smears, it is appropriate to discontinue screenings, and the American Cancer Society suggests stopping pap smears after age 70. If a woman has had a total hysterectomy—removal of uterus, ovaries, and cervix—she does not need to be screened for cervical cancer. However, if she is unsure she has had a total hysterectomy, she should continue to have cervical screenings.

Cervical Cancer Screening

Because pap smears test for *precancerous* lesions, the goal is to catch cervical cancer before it occurs. When caught early, cervical cancer can be 100 percent curable. Some studies have shown that pap smears decrease cervical cancer mortality by about 50 percent.

Colon Cancer Screening

You can beat the odds of developing a very common cancer by getting appropriate colon cancer screening. The lifetime incidence of colon cancer is around 1 in 10, and colorectal cancer is the second leading cause of death from cancer in the United States.

More than 90 percent of people diagnosed with colon cancer are 50 or older, and the average age of diagnosis is 64. Furthermore, research indicates that by age 50, one in four people has polyps—and some of these may be precancerous. Colon cancer is very treatable at early stages, so arm yourself with knowledge on how to screen for this very preventable cancer.

Risk factors for colon cancer include:

◆ Being over age 50

◆ Having a personal history of colorectal cancer

◆ Polyps in the colon or rectum

◆ Ovarian, endometrial, or breast cancer

◆ Ulcerative colitis or Crohn's disease

◆ A parent, brother, sister, or child with colorectal cancer or polyps

◆ Certain hereditary conditions, such as familial adenomatous polyposis (FAP) and hereditary nonpolyposis colon cancer (HNPCC; Lynch Syndrome)

There are several methods for conducting a colon screening. Here's a look at what's currently available and also what's on the horizon.

Fecal Occult Blood Test

If you notice bright red blood in your stool, you're obviously going to consult your physician about what this means. Colon cancer, however, frequently does not show up as overt blood; it may just present as miniscule amounts of blood that are not visible to the naked eye. A fecal occult blood test is a test to check stool for blood that can only be seen with a microscope. In this test, small samples of stool are placed on special cards and returned to the doctor or laboratory for testing. A positive fecal occult blood test may be a sign of polyps or cancer.

Sigmoidoscopy

Sigmoidoscopy is a procedure to look inside the rectum and lower (sigmoid) colon for polyps, abnormal areas, or cancer. A thin, tubelike instrument with a light and a lens for viewing—called a sigmoidoscope—is inserted through the rectum into the sigmoid colon. A sigmoidoscopy and a digital rectal exam (DRE) may be used together to screen for colorectal cancer.

Longevity Facts _____

Sigmoidoscopy screening reduces the risk of death by 59 percent for cancers within reach of the sigmoidoscope. Stool blood cards have been shown to reduce the risk of death from colorectal cancer by 15 percent to 33 percent. And patients screening with a colonoscopy have a 58 percent reduction in incidence of colon cancer and a 61 percent reduction in death from colon cancer.

Digital Rectal Exam

A digital rectal exam (DRE) may be a part of the yearly physical exam. The doctor or nurse inserts a lubricated, gloved finger into the lower part of the rectum to feel for lumps or anything else that seems unusual.

Barium Enema

A barium enema is material used to highlight structures during x-rays of the lower gastrointestinal tract. A chalky liquid that contains barium is put into the rectum. The barium coats the lower gastrointestinal tract and x-rays are taken. This procedure, also called a lower GI series, can detect masses or polyps in the colon.

Colonoscopy

Colonoscopy is a procedure to look inside the rectum and colon for polyps, abnormal areas, or cancer. A colonoscope is inserted through the rectum into the colon. A colonoscope is a thin, tubelike instrument with a light and a lens for viewing. It may also have a tool to remove polyps or tissue samples, which are checked under a microscope for signs of cancer.

New screening tests being studied in clinical trials include virtual colonoscopy and a DNA stool test. Virtual colonoscopy is a procedure that uses CT (computer tomography) to make a series of pictures of the colon. The computer then puts the pictures together to create detailed images that may show polyps and other abnormalities on the inside surface of the colon. The DNA stool test checks DNA in stool cells for genetic changes that may be a sign of colorectal cancer.

Doctors' Orders

Despite numerous anecdotal claims, there is no evidence-based data showing that colon cleansing has any benefit for preventing any specific diseases. The colon is meant to hold waste, and it does the job very well. You can maintain colon health by eating plenty of fruits and vegetables (5 to 10 servings a day) and optimizing the fiber in your diet. Increasing your fluid intake when you increase your fiber is important to prevent constipation. Keeping physically active also helps colonic activity.

Hearing Exams

It is estimated that 30 million adults in the United States have hearing loss, and over a third of these cases are noise-induced. While hearing loss does not necessarily impact the life span, it certainly does significantly impact the health span. The National Institutes of Health has a valuable questionnaire that can help you determine if you have signs of hearing loss:

◆ Do you have difficulty hearing over the phone?

◆ Do you have problems hearing two or more people talking at the same time?

◆ Do you turn the TV volume up too high (meaning that others want to turn it down)?

◆ Do you strain to understand conversation?

◆ Do you have trouble hearing in a noisy background?

◆ Do you ask people to repeat themselves?

◆ Do other people seem to mumble?

◆ Do you misunderstand what others say and respond inappropriately?

◆ Do you have trouble understanding the speech of women and children?

◆ Do people get annoyed because you misunderstand what they say?

If you answer yes to three or more of these questions, you may want to consult with your doctor to see if you need an audiometric evaluation to check for possible hearing loss. An audiometric evaluation consists of a series of tests (conducted by a licensed clinical audiologist) to discover how well you hear, as well as to detect any conditions or abnormalities that may affect your hearing or your balance.

Are you at risk for noise-induced hearing loss (NIHL)? NIHL happens when a person is exposed to repetitive loud noises over a period of time. Prolonged noise exposure to sounds over 85 decibels can cause hearing loss. Here are some decibel measures:

◆ *70 decibels:* Normal conversation

◆ *85 decibels:* Heavy city traffic

◆ *95 decibels:* Motorcycle

- *105 decibels:* Personal stereo system at high; aerobics studio stereo volume at health club

- *110 decibels:* Rock concert; 100-watt car stereo

Listening to a personal stereo system at over 60 percent maximum volume over one hour a day can permanently damage hearing.

Tests of Possibly Dubious Merit

While certain tests and screenings have obvious merit, other tests and screenings are more controversial. Some of these are fads that catch the media's fancy. Others are promoted commercially by the facilities that provide them. And some may indeed be beneficial in certain circumstances. As always, it is recommended that you discuss appropriate screenings with your physician, based on your personal medical history.

Prostate Screening

There is no clear-cut evidence that screening for prostate cancer increases your life span. Deaths from prostate cancer normally occur at an advanced age, so the data on whether treating prostate cancer will lead to decreased mortality is unclear.

Whole Body CT Scans

Commuted Tomography scans—or CT scans—are x-rays that are targeted through the body and provide a cross-sectional picture through the body and can detect internal features such as soft tissue, bone, and blood vessels. Whole body CT scans are CT scans that are taken of the entire body. CT scans are good radiologic procedures for examining the pelvis, abdomen, chest, brain, and spine. They are used to detect size and location of tumors and to evaluate abscesses, inflammation, abdominal aneurysms, kidney stones, and other medical problems.

Over the last few years, there has been quite an interest in whole body CT scans by consumers interested in pursuing the fountain of youth. This has been, in part, due to heavy marketing by facilities offering these scans. Whole body CT scans are touted as early detection techniques for cancers and other diseases in healthy, asymptomatic individuals. But do they help promote longevity? Probably not.

Besides increased radiation exposure, whole body CT scans may produce "false positive" results. Around 80 percent of the abnormalities found in whole body CT scans
are harmless findings, but that can lead to expensive and sometimes invasive workups.
Another drawback is that a normal whole body CT may give a false sense of reassur-
ance to individuals who may then forgo lifestyle measures needed to ensure good
health. It may also cause them to hold off on recommended health screenings that
may catch other health abnormalities.

What is the official government stance on whole body CT scans? The FDA states,
"At this time the FDA knows of no data demonstrating that whole body CT screening is effective in detecting any particular disease early enough for the disease to be
managed, treated, or cured, and advantageously spare a person at least some of the
detriment associated with illness or premature death."

Saliva Tests

Can testing your spit save your life? Maybe, maybe not. The average human produces about 2 pints of saliva a day. This saliva is mostly water, but it also contains
electrolytes, minerals, antibodies, hormones, enzymes, and proteins. The mouth also
contains millions of microorganisms. For these reasons, many tests are ordered on
saliva to check for various diseases in the body. Some of them are recommended by
the FDA, and some have little scientific merit.

Saliva tests for HIV have been approved by the FDA. Similarly, saliva tests for preterm labor and for recurrent breast cancer may have medical merit—definitive
guidelines have not yet been established on the latter two.

Saliva tests offered online and by some (alternative) health providers may test for hormone levels, drug levels, antibodies, and certain cancers. Most of these are not FDA
approved or standardized. These tests can also hurt your pocketbook, as they generally are not covered by insurance.

Stool Tests

Some stool tests have merit—these include the yearly fecal occult blood test that may be done after the age of 50. Other stool tests commonly used in medical practice are stool cultures for various bacterial infections to determine the cause of certain diarrheal illnesses, as well as to check for parasitic infections.

Stool tests are sometimes touted for diagnosing certain toxins and nutritional deficiencies. There is no scientific evidence to back most of these claims.

Antioxidant Levels

Antioxidants such as vitamin E, vitamin C, and beta-carotene play a role in aging and disease, but just how much is under scientific debate. Certain practitioners advertise ways to check antioxidant levels, including laser scanners to check for deficiencies in antioxidants in the body. Laser scanners may be able to check for beta-carotenes, but not much else. Antioxidant testing kits are also available over the Internet but are not really reliable and are not FDA approved.

> **Words to the Wise**
>
> Most people who eat a balanced diet are probably not deficient in antioxidants. Optimizing fruits and vegetables high in antioxidants, rather than spending hundreds of dollars on dubious testing or supplements, is probably a more reliable way to ensure antioxidant deficiencies do not exist.

United States Preventive Services Task Force Recommendations

The best way to ensure your longevity is to make sure you have followed up on what is recommended for your age, gender, and personal risk factors. Sounds simple, but over 50 percent of adults do not do so and thus miss golden opportunities to prolong their lives.

The United States Preventive Services Task Force (USPSTF) division of the government has compiled a list of screenings shown to have value in increasing health in individuals. The recommendations, along with some explanations, are discussed in the following sections.

Recommendations for Men

Abdominal aneurysm screening is recommended for men age 65 to 75 who have ever smoked.

Recommendations for Women

Women with a high risk of breast cancer should discuss medication therapy called chemoprevention with their doctor. All women aged 40 and over should get periodic mammograms.

Genetic screening for breast and ovarian cancer is recommended in women whose family history includes an increased risk for specific genetic mutations called BRCA1 and BRCA2.

Osteoporosis screening is recommended in post-menopausal women aged 65 and older and in women aged 60 and older with an increased risk for fractures.

Recommendations for Men and Women

Some medical conditions obviously can affect both men and women, and there are specific screenings and tests for these conditions. These include:

- Colon cancer screening is recommended every 5 to 10 years after the age of 50.
- Regular high blood pressure screenings at the yearly physical or office visit.
- Diabetes screening for adults with high blood pressure or high cholesterol.
- Alcohol misuse screening.

Doctors' Orders _____

Do you have a potential alcohol problem? Two or more yes responses to the following questions mean you need to discuss this further with your physician:

- Have you ever felt you should cut down on your drinking?
- Have people annoyed you by criticizing your drinking?
- Have you ever felt bad or guilty about your drinking?
- Have you ever had a drink first thing in the morning to steady your nerves or get rid of a hangover (or as an "eye-opener")?

- ◆ Cholesterol screening is recommended for men aged 35 and older and women aged 45 and older. The cholesterol measurement should include total cholesterol and HDL (high density lipoprotein) cholesterol.

- ◆ Obesity screening as appropriate. This generally includes the weight and body mass index; it can also include the waist measurement.

HIV/AIDS and STD Screening Recommendations

Syphilis screening is recommended for all high-risk people. HIV screening is recommended for all adults at increased risk for HIV. People at high risk for HIV include those who have injected drugs or steroids or shared equipment (such as needles or syringes) with others.

This category also includes those who have had unprotected vaginal, anal, or oral sex with men who have sex with men, multiple partners, or anonymous partners; those who have exchanged in sex for drugs or money; and those who have been diagnosed with or treated for hepatitis, tuberculosis (TB), or a sexually transmitted disease (STD), such as syphilis. This also includes those who have had unprotected sex with someone who fits into any of the preceding categories.

Doctors' Orders

The EIA (enzyme immunoassay), which is collected from blood drawn from a vein, is the most common screening test used to look for antibodies to HIV. A positive (reactive) EIA should be followed up with a confirmatory test, such as the Western blot, to make a positive diagnosis. There are EIA tests that use other body fluids to look for antibodies to HIV. These include oral fluid tests and urine tests. Oral fluid tests use saliva collected from the mouth, using a special collection device. This is an EIA antibody test similar to the standard blood EIA test. A follow-up confirmatory Western blot uses the same oral fluid sample. Urine tests use urine instead of blood. The sensitivity and specificity, and thereby the accuracy, of urine tests are less than that of the blood and oral fluid tests.

Tobacco Use Screening

Doctors should ask their patients whether they smoke and provide tools to help them quit smoking, if they do. *Quitting smoking is the single most important lifestyle measure you can do to increase your overall longevity.*

Most smokers or former smokers are curious about whether they should get routine screening for lung cancer. It is well known that smoking greatly increases the risk for lung cancer. The surprising answer is that no benefits have been established for screening for lung cancer in people without symptoms. This includes high-risk people such as smokers or ex-smokers. However, any lung problem, such as an unremitting cough or blood in the sputum, should be worked up appropriately—this may include a chest x-ray.

Longevity Facts _____

New research published in the *New England Journal of Medicine*, by scientists with the famous Framingham Heart Study, found that the standard risk factors—high blood pressure, high cholesterol, family history, advanced age, smoking, obesity, lack of exercise, and diabetes—proved to be just as accurate when it came to predicting heart disease as intensive special testing.

Healing Quickly from Surgery

You will probably undergo a surgical procedure at some point in your life. In many instances, the condition requiring surgery was identified by a routine test or screening. Ensuring that you do not have complications before and after a surgical procedure is essential to both your health span and your life span.

The nice thing about elective surgery is that so much is under your control. For starters, follow all the pre-op and post-op guidelines your surgeon gives you for your particular surgery. In addition, there are other measures you can take to promote optimal healing. If some of these are lifestyle changes for you, consider making them permanent!

Two weeks before surgery:

◆ Don't smoke.

◆ Don't drink.

◆ Avoid excessive stress or exertion. (Don't pull all-nighters getting that last-minute project for work done, and don't choose this time to run the half-marathon.)

◆ Avoid people who are obviously ill.

◆ Contact your doctor if you have any change in health status, including colds or infections.

- Try to sleep eight hours a night.

- Be careful of medications that may increase bruising or bleeding—you usually want to avoid ibuprofen or medications in that category. Acetaminophen is generally fine for aches and pains. Be sure to discuss medications with your doctor before the surgery.

- Tell your doctor about any herbs and supplements you are taking, as some can interfere with the surgery or increase bruising. Most guidelines suggest stopping all supplements and herbs at least two weeks prior to an elective surgery.

Two weeks after surgery, in addition to the recommendations listed previously:

- Listen to your body. Rest if you're tired, and avoid exertion if it hurts excessively. You probably need more down time than you think you do. However, try to be appropriately active—getting up and about helps prevent blood clots, and excessive resting can make you more tired and lead to muscle weakness.

- Slowly progress your diet—it takes a few days for your gastrointestinal tract to catch up after any surgery, and small meals taken frequently will help your digestion.

- Be mindful when taking pain medications. Take medications as prescribed by your doctor to keep yourself comfortable.

- Avoid excessively salty, greasy, or over-processed foods.

- Practice deep breathing for at least 10 minutes a day after surgery—this helps prevent atelectatis (stiff lungs) and helps clear secretions, as well as reduce your blood pressure and stress.

- Practice guided imagery. Think healthy thoughts—focus your energies on the part of your body that is recuperating and send positive energy to the healing area.

- Practice patience. Your body has its natural rhythms and will heal on its own time. Frustration generally arises out of expectations that are unrealistic, given the body's natural healing state.

And as always, think about what is going right in your life, what you want to create, and what is working. Your body will thank you.

In the end, to live a long and healthy life, you want to make sure you are getting screened for preventable diseases. You may end up adding years to your life this way.

And for foreseeable medical events such as surgeries—you can avoid adverse events by a little foresight and preplanning. It's easy to plan for a long life—so much is in your hands!

The Least You Need to Know

◆ There are certain screening tests that have been proven to increase your longevity. These include breast screening, pap smears, and colon screening.

◆ Whole body CT scans may harm you more than they help.

◆ Saliva tests and antioxidant levels may be questionable in diagnosis of medical disorders.

◆ Find out if you need any special tests based on your personal risk factors by reviewing the United States Preventive Task Force recommendations.

◆ Live longer by learning how to avoid complications and heal from any surgeries that you have.

Part 2

The Longevity Lifestyle

How do you live, sleep, eat, and play to live a long, healthy life? Adopting a longevity lifestyle, no matter what your age, can help you in your quest for vitality throughout your life. In this part, we broaden our look at keeping your body vibrantly healthy. You take a quick refresher course on the benefits of exercise, healthy sleep, and sex, and learn which vitamins and supplements are really worth your while. You also discover which foods and diets are scientifically proven to prolong your life span and optimize your health span, and understand how your weight plays into your health. Pulling it all together, you walk away with a personalized program of a longevity lifestyle—one that makes sense to you—and obtain a knowledge of how optimizing your lifestyle pays dividends in prolonging your longevity.

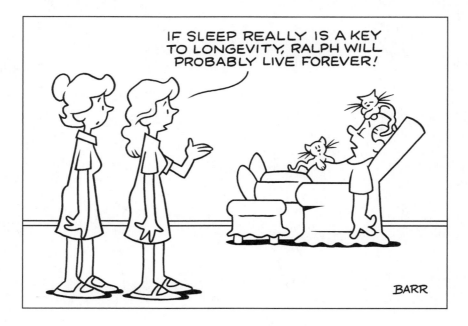

Chapter 4

Nutrition for Life

In This Chapter

◆ Good nutrition and longevity

◆ Colorful is healthful

◆ The lowdown on fat, protein, and salt

◆ Understanding glycemics

◆ Is organic food worth the price?

◆ Stocking your healthy pantry

Making good nutritional choices is an essential component of the longevity lifestyle. Your body needs fuel to perform optimally over the course of your life span. Choose the right fuels, and your body is primed for peak performance.

Good nutrition sets the stage for great health now and for your golden years as well. The food you eat is a feast of substances, helping to orchestrate all the complex biochemical reactions in the cells of your body. A healthy feast ensures that your cells are humming and happy. An unhealthy feast, however, sets you up for chronic diseases down the pike that limit your longevity and reduce the quality of your life. What's an unhealthy feast? It's one with a chronic lack of healthy nutrients, especially plant nutrients, coupled with an intake of unhealthy foods, especially high-fat fast foods.

A Dangerous Legacy

While life expectancy has doubled in the past 200 years—largely because of improvements in sanitation, reduction in infectious diseases, and reduction of infant/mother mortality—the incidence of chronic debilitating disease has skyrocketed. And if we don't make some changes *now*, it is estimated that future generations will, for the first time in history, have shortened life expectancy. This is not a good legacy to leave our children and grandchildren.

There are several reasons for this situation:

- Our intake of whole, unprocessed healthy foods, especially plant foods, is being replaced by processed, often nutrient-deficient foods.

- Our lives are becoming largely sedentary, due to automobiles and other labor-saving devices.

- As a society, we are becoming increasingly obese.

- Social isolation and depression also play a role.

Doctors' Orders _____

Don't eat anything your great-grandmother wouldn't recognize as food. Think about that when you pick up that tube of Go-Gurt. Would she know how to administer that?

—Michael Pollan, author of *The Omnivore's Dilemma,* on choosing wholesome, nutritious foods (fourth annual Nutrition and Health conference, San Diego, May 2007)

Studies of the food habits of people in different countries, especially when compared with the way we eat in the United States, usually show that longevity is linked to the consumption of a plant-based diet high in fruits, vegetables, whole grains, legumes, and fiber, and low in animal fat and animal protein.

Scientific studies during the 1960s and 1970s found relationships between food consumption and chronic disease. These findings contradicted the belief that the United States was the best-fed nation in the world. We are over-fed, not well-fed. When fast food entered the picture, our eating habits changed, and so did our health.

Most health experts now recommend that we eat at least 5 servings of fruits and vegetables per day; 8 to 13 servings may be even more ideal, depending on your total caloric needs.

◆ One serving of fruit is a medium-sized piece of whole fruit (approximately the size of a tennis ball), $\frac{1}{2}$ cup of cut-up fruit, or $\frac{1}{4}$ cup of dried fruit.

◆ One serving of veggies includes 2 cups of raw leafy greens, $\frac{1}{2}$ cup of cooked vegetables, or 1 medium carrot.

◆ One serving of grains includes 1 slice of bread, $\frac{1}{2}$ cup of hot cereal, or 1 ounce of ready-to-eat cereal.

◆ One serving of milk is 1 cup.

◆ One serving of protein includes 2 to 3 ounces of meat/poultry/fish, 1 cup of beans, 1 large egg, $\frac{1}{3}$ cup of nuts, or $\frac{1}{4}$ cup of seeds.

Easier Than You Think

Every three years or so, a whole new crop of nutrition and diet books is launched on the public. How to choose what's nutritionally sound can be an overwhelming task. With the all-fruit diet, the raw diet, the sugar addict's diet, and the south of whatever diet, how is a concerned consumer to know what evidence exists that they work, and even more importantly, that they won't do any harm? The truth is, juicy books sell, even if there's not a lot of science to back them up. And to make matters worse, the scientific evidence seems to change every time you look in the newspaper. Here are some basic principles you can follow that will probably stand the test of time:

◆ Choose whole, unprocessed foods whenever you can.

◆ Eat as much produce as you can; aim for at least 5 to 10 servings of fruits and veggies every day. Vegetable juice is acceptable, but fruit juice may aggravate obesity and diabetes, so eating fruits in their natural state is the preferable way to go.

◆ Limit your intake of animal food—beef, pork, lamb, dairy, and poultry. Go for the low-fat varieties whenever possible. Substitute fish or vegetable protein when you can.

◆ Eat 1 to 2 servings of whole grains at every meal.

◆ Eat 1 to 2 servings of raw or toasted nuts per day (without added fat and salt).

def•i•ni•tion

Legumes are the fruits or seeds of plants such as beans, peas, and lentils.

◆ Eat 1 to 3 servings of *legumes* per day.

◆ Use extra-virgin olive oil or canola oil for cooking.

◆ Be sure that any canned, boxed, or frozen processed foods are limited in fat, sugar, and sodium.

Understanding the Food/Longevity Connection

Specific food groups have an impact on your health and longevity. Foods are roughly broken down into three categories: fats, carbohydrates, and proteins. These categories are known as the macronutrients, or nutrients that you can see, such as the muscle protein of that chicken leg, or the marbled fat on your steak. Micronutrients, on the other hand, are the vitamins, minerals, and other healthy substances in our foods that we can't see but that are essential for our health and longevity.

Macronutrients

Why are macronutrients so important? Let's take a closer look.

◆ Fats are a major source of energy and provide building blocks for healthy cell membranes, hormones, and neurotransmitters in the brain. They also provide a vehicle for the absorption of the fat-soluble vitamins: A, D, E, and K. Fat also adds flavor and sensual enjoyment to food.

◆ Carbohydrates are our main source of energy and also provide much of our fiber, along with vitamins and minerals.

◆ Proteins are needed to build healthy internal organs, bones, muscles, and skin, as well as our hair, nails, and teeth. Proteins also make up most of the hormones, antibodies, and enzymes that are needed to keep biologic processes going. Finally, protein foods (and carbs!) are also sources of vitamins and minerals.

Micronutrients

Micronutrients are the vitamins, minerals, *phytochemicals*, and other health-enhancing substances in whole foods that are not visible to the naked eye. All of these nutrients are essential to good health.

Let's start with some important micro-nutrients—the phytochemicals. Fruits and vegetables are loaded with these, and we have only recently begun to identify and understand the critical role they play in our good health. In this investigation, color is king.

def•i•ni•tion

Phytochemicals are chemical compounds found in plant food; the phytochemicals in the plants we *eat* are referred to as phytonutrients.

What Color Is Your Diet?

Fruits and veggies are colorful and beautiful. They have eye appeal! Perhaps this is why Mother Nature created beauty in the plant world, so we would be drawn to eating these health-enhancing foods. What would look more appealing on a white dinner plate—a pile of bland-looking white food or a tantalizing array of beautifully colored fruits and vegetables?

Fruits and vegetables, in addition to being high in vitamins, minerals, and fiber, are loaded with antioxidants and other compounds, such as polyphenols, that protect against chronic disease, including heart disease, diabetes, and cancer. The USDA fruit and veggie campaign has emphasized "Eat 5 to Stay Alive," but push your fruit and vegetable intake to 8 or 10 servings or more per day—that means 2 or 3 per meal, plus another 1 or 2 for snacks—and you're on your way!

When it comes to fruits and veggies, color is primo! Color in produce is an indicator of high quantities of antioxidants, polyphenols, and other protective chemicals. Free radicals can damage the DNA in your cells and increase your risk of cancer, but foods rich in nature's own protective chemicals should be your first line of defense.

What do your food colors indicate? The deep color of fruits and veggies often indicate these foods are high in the carotenes, a huge collection of over 500 chemicals, of which about 50 can be converted into vitamin A in the body. The most common carotenes include alpha- and beta-carotene, beta-cryptoxanthin, lycopene, lutein, and zeaxanthin.

Carotenes and vitamin A are important for a healthy immune system, as well as for healthy vision and cell growth. Carotenes also function as antioxidants and are felt to protect against a number of cancers. One recent study also suggested that people with higher blood levels of beta-carotene had a lower risk of cognitive (intellectual) decline.

Green plants (especially spinach, collard and mustard greens, kale, parsley, avocado, and green peas) and yellow corn contain beta-carotene, as well as the carotenes lutein and zeaxanthin. These help to prevent cataracts, macular degeneration, osteoporosis, and stroke.

Orange produce such as sweet potatoes/yams, carrots, mangos, cantaloupe, and squash contain alpha- and beta-carotene, both plant precursors to vitamin A. Non-orange produce, such as kale, spinach, chard, parsley, and red peppers, are also high in beta-carotene. (The orange pigment in these foods is covered up by the other pigments in the food.)

B-cryptoxanthin is a carotene found in oranges, tangerines, peaches, nectarines, and papaya. It's also converted into vitamin A in the body and is an antioxidant as well.

What about reducing your risk of cancer? Green cruciferous veggies in particular, such as broccoli, Brussels sprouts, and cabbage, contain cancer-preventing chemicals called indoles, sulforaphane, and isothiocyanate. Don't miss 'em!

> ### Words to the Wise
>
> Try this healthy recipe for a Longevity Smoothie:
>
> ½ cup frozen mixed dark berries
>
> ½ cup frozen mixed tropical fruit
>
> 1 medium ripe banana
>
> 1 cup orange juice
>
> 1 scoop dried soy protein powder
>
> Put everything in a blender and whirl until smooth; add more or less juice to adjust thickness.

Red, purple, and blue fruits and veggies such as berries, grapes, red apples, beets, and red wine are loaded with anthocyanins, nature's antioxidants. These combat inflammation, arthritis, and vascular disease.

Other reddish fruits such as grapefruit, watermelon, papaya, guava, and tomato contain lycopene, another carotene. Lycopene is the most powerful antioxidant in the carotene family, more potent than vitamin E.

Light green plants—celery, pears, garlic, onions—contain quercetin. (Many other plants also contain quercetin, including apples, red grapes, citrus, leafy greens, and berries.) Quercetin is a powerful antioxidant and anti-inflammatory phytochemical that may help to prevent allergies, asthma, cataracts, heart disease, and cancer. Plants in the garlic family also contain allicin, a chemical that helps to reduce blood pressure, fight infections, and also protect against cancer.

Eating lots of colorful produce is one of the best things you can do to enhance your health and keep your body young and fit. Fruits and veggies with the deepest pigment tend to have the most carotenoids, so stock up on color!

What should you look for when choosing fresh fruits and vegetables? Fresh-picked is best; farmers markets often provide produce that was just picked from the fields. Frozen food is an excellent alternative, as those foods are generally processed as soon as they are harvested, locking in the nutrients.

Here are some tips for getting those 5 to 10 servings per day:

◆ Have a fruit smoothie in the morning.

◆ Throw dried or fresh blueberries and/or raisins on your oatmeal every day.

◆ Buy or make up individual packets of veggies, such as carrots and pea pods, and take two or three with you to work every day.

◆ Keep dried fruit at your desk and in your car.

◆ Bring a big salad to school or work with you every day.

◆ Put out a plate of raw veggies to snack on before dinner.

◆ Include at least one fruit and two veggies with every meal.

◆ If you snack between meals, always eat fruit or veggies before you allow yourself anything else.

The Skinny on Fat

In the 1960s and 1970s, doctors thought that animal fats such as butter and red meat were the culprits behind our epidemic of heart disease, so health experts advocated a low animal fat diet. We were advised to reach for margarine instead of butter and ease up on the red meat. Then came the low-fat, high-carb craze, and we loaded up on calorie-laden white flour and white sugar. We also became fatter and fatter, *and* cardiovascular disease remained the number-one killer of Americans. On top of that, researchers discovered that margarine, which was loaded with *trans fat*, was worse for your arteries than butter. Not only did it raise your LDL (bad) cholesterol like butter, but it also lowered your protective HDL (good) cholesterol, and probably caused inflammation.

def•i•ni•tion

A **trans fat** (hydrogenated fat) is a polyunsaturated oil (such as corn oil) that has been turned into a solid fat (such as margarine or vegetable shortening) by exposing it to high heat and pressure. Trans fats became popular because they have a much longer shelf life than butter or liquid oils. Packaged foods made with trans fat, such as cookies and crackers, can sit on store shelves for months without spoiling.

Fats and Inflammation

Why is inflammation such a concern now? Inflammation, aggravated by our current intake of fats and other foods, is felt to be at the root of many degenerative diseases that Americans now face. If you want to prevent chronic, degenerative diseases—including heart disease, Alzheimer's, and perhaps even cancer—you've got to understand a bit about how fats can cause inflammation in our bodies. But first, a few more facts on fats.

Good and Bad Fats

Fats are generally categorized as polyunsaturated, monounsaturated, and saturated:

◆ *Polyunsaturated* fatty acids are usually liquid at room temperature; they include most of the oils seen commonly in the grocery store, including corn, safflower, and soybean oil (omega-6 oils). They also include oils found in fish, nuts, and leafy greens (omega-3 oils). These oils are also used to make trans fats.

◆ *Monounsaturated* fatty acids are also usually liquid at room temperature and include olive, canola, and peanut oil; avocados also contain monounsaturated fats. These fatty acids are also called omega-9 acids.

Longevity Facts

Virgin or extra-virgin olive oil is made by simply cold-pressing oil from olives. One study found that men who consumed about 2 tablespoons per day of virgin olive oil increased their blood level of HDL (good) cholesterol more than men who consumed "ordinary" olive oil. They also had less inflammation in their blood.

◆ *Saturated* fatty acids are usually solid at room temperature and include butter and lard; some oils, such as coconut oil, are also saturated.

The omega-3 oils, and sometimes the omega-9s, are sometimes known as the *anti-inflammatory* oils. When these oils are metabolized in the body, they lead to the production of anti-inflammatory chemicals called eicosanoids, protecting blood vessels and tissues from the damage of free radicals and inflammation. Omega-6 oils, especially those that have been converted into margarines (trans fats), have the opposite effect—they tend to produce more inflammatory chemicals. Naturally saturated fats, such as those found in meats and dairy products, also tip the balance toward inflammation.

The other two classes of lipids in the diet are the sterols (cholesterol and similar compounds) and the phospholipids. Your blood cholesterol levels reflect the amount and types of all of these fats you eat. In addition, some folks are really good at manufacturing some of these for themselves, including cholesterol. You'll read more about these in Chapter 10.

Primitive people probably ate a ratio of omega-6 to omega-3 fats that ranged from 1:1 to about 4:1. Today, scientists estimate our ratio is anywhere from 12 to 20:1. It's not hard to see why. Supermarket shelves are filled with thousands of processed and packaged foods containing hydrogenated and partially hydrogenated trans fats.

This huge intake of inflammatory trans fat, coupled with our reduced intake of omega-3 oils (fish, walnuts, greens) and the resulting imbalance between pro-inflammatory and anti-inflammatory foods, has become severe. This is felt to be a driver behind inflammatory degenerative diseases in the West.

Longevity Facts

Want to live a long and healthy life? Then follow the example of people eating the traditional Mediterranean, Chinese, and Japanese diets—high in plant food and omega-3 fats, and low in meat and processed foods (yes, that means no trans fats!). People from these parts of the world have a leg up on longevity.

Is *all* inflammation bad? No, of course not! Some inflammation is essential; it fires up the healing process and helps to fight off infection. Then, once the job is done, nature steps in again to cool things down with her antioxidants, bringing everything back into balance. Too much inflammation, though, especially chronic inflammation, overwhelms those delicate balance mechanisms and ultimately leads to wear, tear, tissue breakdown, and a shortened life span.

The Glycemic Goof-Up

Carbohydrates are the main source of energy in our diets and are divided into complex and simple carbohydrates. Complex carbohydrates (starches) come from plant foods such as grains, vegetables, beans, and seeds. Simple carbohydrates include sugars, honey, syrups, and the sugar found in fruits.

Carbohydrates, or "carbs" as they have come to be known, have gotten a bad rap recently. Until the turn of the last century, we ate unprocessed carbs; there was no such thing as white flour and white sugar. When the refining of grains began, these "processed," more expensive carbs became a status symbol; for a time, only the wealthy could afford them. The efficiency of mechanization, as well as the growth of the middle class after World War II, led to the widespread use of these foods, and they gradually began to replace healthier whole grain carbs in the American diet.

There are several reasons why whole or unrefined carbs are so much better for you than their white cousins:

◆ They have lots of fiber (good for your bowels).

◆ They contain healthy oils and vitamin E (a natural antioxidant).

◆ They are loaded with nutrients, including B vitamins (good for your heart, brain, and cancer prevention).

Explaining Glycemic

If you read the newspapers or watch the news on TV, you've probably heard the term *glycemic index*. Glycemic literally means "causing sugar (glucose) in the blood." The glycemic index refers to how quickly a particular food, especially a carb, is absorbed and converted into sugar in the bloodstream. A refined carb, such as table sugar, will get absorbed quickly from your intestines, while the sugar in an apple might take a little longer, because your body first has to break down the apple tissue before the fruit sugar is released. Rapid absorption of sugar also means rapid spikes in your insulin secretion, needed to help clear sugar from your blood. These spikes trigger hunger for more intensely sweet food, and the cycle begins again. This persistent cycle can lead to food cravings, weight gain, diabetes, and abnormal cholesterol—not good for your longevity!

Bottom line? Choose whole grain carbs whenever you can!

Fabulous Fiber

Fiber is nondigestible carbohydrate that stays in your gut, keeps your stools soft, keeps food moving efficiently through your GI tract, and reduces blood cholesterol. Fiber also slows down digestion and reduces those spikes of insulin secretion. Finally, it fills you up more than refined foods, creating more satiety and reducing overeating and weight gain. What could be better than this, right? But wait—there's more! The fibrous portions of foods are often close to the vitamins, minerals, and other natural substances in foods that keep you healthy and strong. Refining foods and removing the fiber can lead to loss of these nutrients.

The average Westerner eats about 80 percent *less* dietary fiber than someone living 100 years ago. Health experts in the United States now recommend that the average healthy adult get 20 to 35 g (grams) of total fiber per day; some people may need more in order to maintain bowel health and reduce constipation.

Longevity Facts

The top five foods for dietary fiber are ...

◆ Legumes (15 to 19 g fiber per cup).

◆ Wheat bran (17 g per cup).

◆ Prunes (12 g per cup).

◆ Asian pears (10 g each).

◆ Quinoa (9 g per cup).

Powerful, Healthy Protein

Proteins form muscles, bones and organs, enzymes, hormones, antibodies, and other essential compounds in the body. Many people think they need far more protein than they actually do. The average person needs about 0.4 g of protein per pound of body weight per day. This translates to 60 g of protein for a 150-pound woman and 80 g for a 200-pound man. When you consider that 3 ounces of skinned chicken breast has about 26 g of protein, you can see that it's not that hard for most Americans to get their daily requirement. In fact, studies of food intake show that Americans' protein intake is almost always above the recommended amount: women tend to get 58 to 70 g of protein per day, and men 74 to 110 g per day.

People who exercise vigorously, including body builders, do need more calories proportionately than more sedentary folks, and part of this increased calorie requirement includes protein. However, eating more protein than your body actually needs will *not* lead to bigger muscles. Protein foods help to satisfy hunger and increase a sense of satiety, even more than fat does. Even when you eat a low-calorie diet, if you eat enough protein, you are more likely to feel satiated and not overeat. Studies in numerous countries have shown that when people eat a high-protein breakfast or lunch, they feel more satisfied and tend to eat less at their next meal. Different protein foods create different levels of satiety. One study showed that fish was better at this than beef, chicken, or pork (and you get those healthy fish oils to boot!).

If you take in more than you need of any food, including protein, it is converted to storage fuel (fat). There is also concern that very high–animal protein diets may increase the risk of osteoporosis (brittle bones). This is because the breakdown of animal proteins in the body produces acids that need to be neutralized, and calcium may be pulled from the bones to accomplish this, leading to bone loss. In addition, plant foods containing vitamin K and potassium are important for bone health, and high-protein diets often crowd out these important foods. Excess protein can also put a strain on your kidneys.

People who consume higher levels of protein, especially low-fat or plant-based proteins, seem to have lower blood pressure. One of the amino acids in protein, arginine, is converted in the body to nitrous oxide, which relaxes blood vessels, which in turn can lower blood pressure.

Shaking the Salt Habit

Many of us are so used to salting everything we eat, that we crave it daily; foods without salt often taste bland. Salt is on the FDA's Generally Recognized As Safe list (GRAS); this means that the food industry is not limited in how much salt it can add to processed foods. (See www.fda.gov for more information.) Yet salt is anything but safe; excessive sodium consumption is directly related to elevated blood pressure or hypertension, which is felt to be the cause of 8 million deaths worldwide every year.

A lower salt intake will keep your blood pressure healthy, lowering your risk of heart attack, congestive heart failure, kidney failure, and stroke. Low salt intake is good for your bones, too, reducing your risk of osteoporosis and fractures. Reducing salt intake is a small price to pay for a big longevity payoff.

Putting It All Together

Most nutritionists agree that the healthiest diet is one in which 10 to 15 percent of calories come from lean protein, 20 to 30 percent from healthy fats (omega-3s and olive oil), and the rest from carbs. Most carbs should be from whole grains, legumes, fruits, and veggies, with a minimum coming from refined sugars. The Mediterranean diet, which includes lots of plant food and fiber and uses olive oil as the primary fat, is now advocated by many health experts. You'll read more about the Mediterranean diet in Chapter 6. (See Appendix B for more information on healthy nutrition.)

Organics—Are They Worth It?

Organics are big business; even major supermarket chains are pushing their own lines of organic foods. Some organic produce has been found to have slightly higher levels of several nutrients, especially vitamin C; however, the data on this is sparse. Organic or not, what's *really* health-enhancing is getting those 5 to 10 servings of fruits and veggies per day, period.

Organic fruits and veggies definitely have fewer pesticide residues than conventionally grown produce. They aren't completely pesticide-free because of contamination in the global environment. Whether or not this increases your longevity or reduces your risk of disease, especially cancer, is not clear. For healthy adults, obesity and poor diet pose far greater risk to health than pesticide residues in food. Pregnant women and young children should avoid pesticides when possible, and most commercial baby foods are felt to be pesticide-free.

The Environmental Working Group (EWG) in Washington, D.C., took the 43 most commonly eaten fruits and veggies in the United States and ranked them according to how many pesticide residues they contained. The EWG estimates that you can reduce your intake of pesticides by about 90 percent if you avoid the 12 most commonly contaminated fruits and veggies, also referred to as the "Dirty Dozen": peaches, apples, sweet bell peppers, celery, nectarines, strawberries, cherries, pears, imported grapes, spinach, lettuce, and potatoes. Go for the organic versions of these!

Conversely, the "Consistently Clean" list includes onions, avocados, sweet corn, pineapples, mango, asparagus, sweet peas, kiwi, bananas, cabbage, broccoli, and papaya.

Stocking Up

Good nutrition is essential for a long, healthy life. Make the decision to eat smart and become knowledgeable about the foods you eat. Once you take the plunge into the pleasure of produce and other good food, you will feel so much better, and this new state of well-being will reinforce your good shopping behavior and keep you going.

The healthy pantry consists of the following:

- *Fruits and veggies in all forms:* Fresh, frozen, canned, and dried—as long as they are unprocessed or minimally processed with minimum to no added salt, sugar, and fat.

- *Whole grains:* All varieties. Try experimenting with oat groats, bulgur, quinoa, and brown rice.

- *Nuts:* Raw or roasted—again without added salt and fat.

- *Pulses:* Lentils, peas, beans, and other legumes.

- *Fish:* Especially wild fish or farmed fish low in toxins.

The Least You Need to Know

◆ For a long and healthy life, eat a healthy diet.

◆ Eat as many fruits and vegetables as you can every day; include lots of different colors in your choices.

◆ Use olive oil and canola oil in place of other fats.

◆ Get at least 20 to 35 g of fiber per day.

◆ Eat lean protein; if you're trying to lose weight, fish may be your best bet for protein food.

Chapter 5

Exercise Essentials

In This Chapter

- ◆ The many benefits of regular exercise
- ◆ Has exercise become obsolete?
- ◆ Finding the right fit
- ◆ Keep moving!
- ◆ Staying the course

The human body was meant to move! It was designed to remain active for the entire course of your life. Why is exercise so important? In addition to burning calories and reducing your risk of weight gain and obesity, exercise keeps your heart and brain healthy. It also energizes you and helps you stay motivated to maintain your healthy lifestyle.

What's in It for You?

As the saying goes, if you could bottle exercise and sell it to the public as a longevity tonic, you'd be a billionaire. There is almost *nothing* you can do to improve your health, well-being, and longevity that's better than regular exercise. And it keeps your brain humming to boot! Study after study has shown that people who exercise regularly reduce their chances of dying from cardiovascular disease and other degenerative diseases by as much as 20 percent or more, even if they cling to some other bad habits such as obesity or poor diet. You don't have to be an Olympic athlete to reap these benefits, either. Moderate exercise, done consistently over time, does the trick.

Reducing Your Chronological Age

Up until the 1980s, conventional wisdom had it that muscle wasting was inevitable as we got older. That theory was disproved when researchers found that people in their 70s, 80s, and even 90s could reverse many signs of aging by building up their strength and muscle mass through weight training. Multiple studies have now shown that you can reduce your chronological age with exercise. Miriam Nelson, Ph.D., at Tufts University was one of the first researchers to demonstrate this and has been a prominent advocate of exercise for the elderly.

> **Longevity Facts** _____
>
> Studies have shown that prolonged bed rest can age us by as much as 20 years! Conversely, regular exercise and physical activity has the capacity to keep us youthful. Exercise is the secret to great health and vitality, especially as we age.

def•i•ni•tion _____

Morbidity is the pattern of disease or illness seen in a population.

Even if you've never exercised before, you can still reap these benefits and become physically fit at any age. What's more, getting active again will increase your balance and reduce your risk of falls and fractures, a big source of *morbidity* and mortality in older folks.

Maintaining Your Weight

Believe it or not, once you hit the ripe old age of 20, your metabolism begins to slow down. For every year after that, you generally need fewer calories to maintain your weight, even if your activity levels remain the same. Then at mid-life, muscle mass really starts to slide and body fat increases. This loss of muscle mass has been called *sarcopenia,* and these changes in the body have been called *usual aging.*

Because muscle burns more fuel than fat tissue, weight-bearing exercise, especially weight training, will help you maintain muscle, burn fuel more efficiently, and avoid that gradual weight gain.

Each of us has a different resting energy expenditure (REE). The REE is the number of calories your heart, brain, and other organs use up every day for their normal metabolism, even if you spend the day in bed. If your REE is high, you'll burn more calories every day, and you're less likely to gain weight. If your REE is low, don't get discouraged! You can increase your calorie output with simple changes—such as standing instead of sitting, for example. Studies have shown that people who stand a lot or who tend to fidget can burn up an extra 300 calories per day, compared to those who don't.

Heart and Brain Health

Exercise is good for your muscles, but what about your other organs? Aerobic exercise is one of the best things you can do for your heart, your blood vessels, and your brain. Exercise can reduce your risk of high blood pressure by 50 percent! If you already have hypertension, exercise will lower your blood pressure and may allow you to reduce the dose of your medications. Exercise also reduces your risk of diabetes, which is a big contributor to heart disease and a shortened life span. Finally, aerobic fitness is associated with improved cognition and may help to prevent Alzheimer's disease.

Immune System Benefits

Exercise can reduce your risk of infections. Numerous studies have shown that people who exercise regularly are less likely to get colds and other infections. This becomes really important because, as we age, our risk of influenza and pneumonia tend to increase.

However, excessive exercise can lead to *immunosuppression;* for example, people who run marathons are more likely to get sick in the one to two weeks after a big run. Numerous supplements, including glutamine, carbohydrates, zinc, and antioxidants, have been tried in an attempt to prevent this immune system change. Of these supplements, carbohydrates are probably the most effective (drink 1 liter of a sports drink per hour of exercise). This seems to reduce the release of stress hormones, including cortisol and epinephrine; it may also reduce the production of inflammatory chemicals in the blood.

def•i•ni•tion

Immunosuppression is the term used for the inhibition of the normal functioning of our infection-fighting white blood cells.

Mother Nature encourages moderation, even in the pursuit of fitness.

Healthy Joints and Bones

Exercise keeps your joints healthy and strong, in part by increasing blood flow to the joints. Exercise also reduces the pain, swelling, and disability that accompany arthritis, including both osteoarthritis and rheumatoid arthritis. Strength training exercise also increases bone and muscle density, especially in women. And as mentioned earlier, regular exercise improves muscle strength and balance, increases the capacity to walk and climb, and reduces the risk of falls and fractures. Did you know that an elderly woman who breaks her hip has a 15 percent chance of dying from complications of her fracture? And 50 percent of women sustaining hip fractures will never walk on their own again.

Lift That Mood!

Exercise can reduce stress, anxiety, and depression. This includes endurance exercise, as well as strength training and even stretching exercises such as those done in yoga. It's not clear if these changes come about because people feel stronger and more empowered when they exercise or because exercise positively impacts neurotransmitters and other chemicals in the brain that affect mood. Studies have shown that formerly depressed people who exercise for at least two and a half to three hours per week are much less likely to have a relapse of depression. Exercise has also been shown to improve sleep in older adults, probably because it reduces stress and relaxes muscles.

Doctors' Orders

Avoid vigorous exercise for at least several hours before bedtime. Being revved up from exercise can make it *harder* to fall asleep.

Other Benefits

Regular exercise can also significantly reduce your risk of colon cancer (by up to 50 percent), diverticular disease, gallstones, and (for men only, of course) prostate enlargement.

Some Exercise Background

It is estimated that prehistoric people walked up to 20 miles per day. When you *had* to rely on your own muscles for locomotion, food production, and other daily activities, you were certain to get a lot more exercise than we do today. When did that all change? The Industrial Revolution and the everyday use of automobiles, especially after World War II, really changed the landscape of exercise and fitness for the average American. The advent of computers and video games has also had an impact, especially for young people. And many schools now do not have any regular physical fitness program, let alone any mandatory exercise requirements for students. Exercise has become obsolete.

Fitness in All Forms

So—how fit are you? If you're not certain, you may want to get an assessment by a fitness trainer. Chances are, if you are over 40 and have also been sedentary, your fitness level will be low and your body fat percentage will be high. The good thing about this is that you will quickly start to see improvements in your numbers, and this quick shift is a great way to inspire yourself to keep going. If you are 40 or older, get a checkup with your doctor before increasing your exertion level.

Doctors' Orders

If you are currently a couch potato, check with your doctor before you start any fitness program, especially if you have …

- A history of heart disease.
- High blood pressure.
- A heart condition or any other vascular disease.
- A family history of diabetes.
- Chest discomfort, faintness, or difficulty breathing during any physical exertion, including sex.
- Persistent or sharp pain in your muscles or joints.
- Any other chronic illness, are pregnant, or are over age 50.

To find a qualified personal trainer, look for someone who's been certified by at least one of the following organizations:

- The American College of Sports Medicine
- The National Academy of Sports Medicine
- The American Council on Exercise
- The Cooper Institute for Aerobics Research

- ◆ The Aerobics and Fitness Association of America
- ◆ The National Strength and Conditioning Association

Aerobic

Aerobic exercise is anything that makes your heart rate increase, gets your blood pumping, and makes you breathe harder. Aerobic exercise is often referred to as endurance exercise. If you're new to this, or if you've slacked off for a while, especially if you're over 40, then start slowly—as little as 5 to 15 minutes per day, gradually working up to at least 30 minutes per day, and ideally 45 to 60 minutes per day. The more you exercise, the more fit you will become. Your goal is to exercise at *moderate to vigorous* intensity. What's moderate? If you feel a little winded, but you can still carry on a conversation, then you're at the moderate level; if you're too winded for a conversation, then you're at the vigorous level. Moderate exercises include walking briskly (at a 3- to 4-mile-per-hour pace), playing doubles tennis, or mowing your lawn. Vigorous exercise includes running, spinning (indoor cycling classes), or playing soccer or a game of basketball.

Another way to do this is to get your heart rate up periodically to 65 to 80 percent of your predicted maximum based on your age, as shown in the following table.

First, calculate your maximum heart rate, which is estimated by subtracting your age from 220. To achieve moderate intensity exercise, your heart rate should be 50 to 70 percent of your maximum heart rate. For example, if you are 50 years old, your maximum heart rate is 170; your 50 percent and 70 percent rates would be 85 to 120 beats per minute. To achieve vigorous intensity exercise, your heart rate should be 70 to 85 percent of your maximum, or 120 to 145.

Percent of Maximum Heart Rate	Age							
	30	40	50	60	70	80	90	100
100	190	180	170	160	150	140	130	120
85	162	153	145	136	128	119	111	102
70	133	126	119	112	105	98	91	84
50	95	90	85	80	75	70	65	60

If you're below 50 percent of your maximum, you're not yet at the point where you're starting to get the benefits of endurance exercise; keep going!

Aerobic exercise is good for your heart, your brain, and your blood vessels. It also lowers blood pressure, reduces body fat (see the following table), and reduces your risk of diabetes. It reduces constipation to boot! Pick any form that works for you—walking, jogging, dancing, hiking, cycling, etc. If you get bored with one, then take up another. If you own a dog, you've got a built-in excuse to walk—get the dog out for at least two (15-minute) walks per day. It'll do you both good!

How much body fat is healthy? Our percent body fat increases as we get older, and our lean body mass (muscle and bone) decreases.

Age	Excellent	Body Fat Good	Fair
For men:			
40–49	Up to 18.1%	18.2–21.1%	21.2–24.1%
50–59	Up to 19.8%	19.9–22.7%	22.8–25.7%
60 and over	Up to 20.3%	20.4–23.5%	23.6–26.7%
For women:			
40–49	Up to 23.5%	23.6–26.4%	26.5–30.1%
50–59	Up to 26.6%	26.7–30.1%	30.2–33.5%
60 and over	Up to 27.5%	27.6–30.9%	31.0–34.3%

Another way to figure out if you're healthy is to calculate your body mass index (BMI); you can do this using a BMI table, or you can divide your weight in kilograms by your height in meters squared. The BMI correlates fairly closely with your body fat percentage, though someone who has very bulky muscles from weight training may have an elevated BMI and low body fat; this is the exception, however.

Measuring your steps as you walk your way to fitness is easy, if you have a pedometer. Your local sports store will have these in stock and you should be able to get one for under $20. Pedometers are like small computers that you clip to your waist, and they measure the number of steps you take. Fitness experts recommend that we walk 10,000 steps per day to achieve and maintain healthy fitness levels. For someone who is in relatively good shape, this will take an average of 75 minutes of walking. If your goal is weight loss, however, you will probably need to *step* this up (no pun intended!) to 12,000 to 15,000 steps per day.

If you want to stick with moderate-intensity exercise, then the current recommendations from the Centers for Disease Control and the American College of Sports Medicine are a *minimum* of 30 minutes on five or more days of the week (60 minutes is probably the ideal). You can divide up the 30 minutes into segments, if that's easier, but each segment should be no less than 10 minutes. If you're a vigorous exerciser, then 20 minutes or more at least three days per week is considered sufficient. And remember—the more you do, the more fit you'll become. Be sure to include warm-up and cool-down periods, including stretching.

Don't overdo it. Going overboard puts you at risk for joint and muscle injuries, especially as you get older. And extreme exercise, as mentioned earlier, can increase your risk of getting sick. While being underweight is generally not a concern for the older crowd, eating disorders are becoming more common in middle-aged women; for these folks, overdoing it on the exercise and weight loss can lead to abnormally low body fat, which increases your risk of osteoporosis and fractures. Finally, focusing on just one sport, such as running, and ignoring other activities, including strength and balance training along with stretching, can also increase your susceptibility to injuries.

Strength

Strength training is also called resistance exercise. Studies in older folks show incredible improvement in muscle strength and muscle mass when people weight train two or three times per week—muscle strength can increase by more than 170 percent! And strength training will help prevent bone loss or osteoporosis. Some studies have even shown that weight training can *increase* bone density. Weight training of a specific set of muscles should never be done on consecutive days; your muscles need a chance to rest and recover for at least 48 hours after a workout.

Any exercise that keeps you on your feet, such as walking and jogging, will help work your bones and improve bone strength. Exercises such as cycling and water aerobics will also help, but are a little less effective than being on your feet. Swimming, which is great for the heart, muscles, and flexibility, gives the least weight-bearing benefit.

As we age, strengthening the muscles in the back and lower extremities is especially important to maintain a healthy gait, stride, and balance, and to reduce falls and fractures. Start out with low weight and do 8 to 15 repetitions of each exercise; when you get to 12 to 15 reps without too much difficulty, then it's time to increase the amount of weight. Take three seconds to lift the weight and three seconds to slowly return to starting position. Exhale as you lift the weight, and inhale as you lower; never hold your breath. Your muscles should feel pleasantly sore with lifting, especially if you are a beginner. If you experience any sharp or unusual pain, including headaches, then stop and consult with a health professional.

Many gyms now offer classes in using exercise balls. Strength training exercises can be done on one of these balls using free weights. Not only do you work your arms and legs, but working on an exercise ball makes your *core muscles* work as well. Pilates is another excellent form of exercise to strengthen your core.

def•i•ni•tion

The **core muscles** are the muscles of the trunk (from the shoulders and spine down to the pelvic floor), that provide stability and help to maintain good posture. Keeping your core muscles in good shape will maintain balance and help to prevent falls as you get older. In addition, core training your pelvic floor muscles will reduce your risk of bladder and bowel incontinence as you get older.

Flexibility

Flexibility exercises, such as those found in tai chi and yoga, have many health benefits, including reducing the aches, pains, and general stiffness that come with age. Yoga has been found to improve numerous health conditions, including depression, stress, anxiety, high blood pressure, and chronic back pain.

Balance

Maintaining balance is crucial, as we get older, in order to avoid falls and fractures. Most of us start to lose our ability to balance once we reach our 40s, though we're usually unaware of it early on. Without attention to exercises that help us to maintain our core muscles and balance, our risk of falling increases with every decade. In fact, about 30 percent of people over the age of 65 will fall at least once every year. Many older Americans become so fearful of falling that they stop exercising altogether— and this reduces strength and balance even further. The good news is that great balance is something we can all maintain, with the appropriate exercises.

To improve your balance …

 ◆ Keep up with your weight-training; studies have shown that lifting weights also improves balance.

♦ Walk and perform endurance exercises to improve both balance and coordination.

♦ Take up tai chi, which has been shown to reduce falls. Yoga balance postures are also great at developing balance.

♦ Learn to stand on your toes. Start out on both feet, then practice one-legged stands.

♦ Stand on your heels, using a wall behind you for support.

♦ Practice balance by standing on one foot whenever you are waiting in a line; just be sure you have something sturdy to hold on to in case you lose your balance!

Words to the Wise

Here's a test to see how well you can balance: stand next to a wall or sturdy chair for support. Then stand on one foot with your arms extended out horizontally to the sides. Now close your eyes. If you are over the age of 40, you should be able to stand without having to move your foot for at least 15 seconds. Having a hard time with this? Don't worry—you're not alone. Keep practicing until you're able to do it on either foot!

Keeping Physically Active

Walking and cycling will keep your body fit and help maintain your weight. For those of you who hate the thought of exercise, however, there are some other ways to burn calories and keep your muscles strong.

Don't Sit Down!

If you've been around children much, you know how teachers are always admonishing them to sit still and pay attention. Well, it turns out that those of us who fidget and have a hard time sitting still burn up on average 300 calories more per day than our slothful comrades. In fact, a study published in 2005 found that the obese folks tended to spend two hours more per day just sitting, compared to their thin counterparts. This adds up to a huge difference in overall calorie expenditure—to the tune of up to 30 pounds of extra weight per year for the couch potatoes.

Our current environment of remote controls and other labor-saving devices tends to discourage activity, but you can learn to become more active. This may take some persistence in making behavioral changes, such as walking more at work, taking the stairs when you can, and standing up more during the day, rather than sitting.

Do What You Love

Exercise doesn't have to mean going to an aerobics class that makes you wince just thinking about it. Do what you love! Do you like to dance? Get outdoors? Hike or garden? There is something for everyone out there! Join a club, go to a dance or Jazzercise class, get a dog, or dust off your bike. Mop the floor to your favorite rock 'n' roll song! Even if it seems like drudgery at first, don't give up! Eventually, you will feel so good from exercise that you will make it a priority in your life.

Dealing with Setbacks

Having a hard time getting started? Or perhaps you suffer from the typical malady—you've got great intentions, you go out and buy that exercise bike, and it ends up becoming a clothes rack in your family room. There are three common reasons why people fail in their attempts at fitness: time, fatigue, and laziness. Here are some suggestions for addressing each.

Time

There are tricks to help you here. Incorporate small portions of exercise into your daily routine, such as a 15-minute walk at lunchtime and after work. Let go of a task that you really didn't want to do anyway, such as serving on yet another committee, and schedule a weight workout instead. Start with one or two workouts per week and when this becomes a habit, then gradually do more. Give yourself 8 to 10 weeks to incorporate your new health habits.

Energy

You may think you don't have the energy for exercise, but once you get started, you'll find that regular exercise gives you *more* energy, not less. Getting blood pumping to your muscles and your brain wakes you up, makes you feel great, and inspires you to do more. You've just got to *start!* With more energy, you may find yourself getting things done more efficiently, freeing up even more time in your day (an added bonus).

Laziness

You're *not* lazy, but you may be listening to the voice of that little saboteur in your head more than you should. The trick here is to keep focusing on your fitness goals when you find yourself wanting to give up.

Keep It Going!

Lots of other things can help keep your motivation up:

◆ Keep a log of your progress. Seeing a visual record of your gradual increases in endurance, strength, and flexibility helps many people keep going. Don't let yourself off the hook if your progress does plateau for a period. Plateaus are common and may simply mean that you're ready for the next level of challenge. This is great news!

◆ Exercise to music you love.

◆ If you're exercising at home, do it while watching your favorite movie or TV show. Don't stop until the show is over.

◆ If you have a hard time getting going, schedule a class or more per week. Commit to getting there on time and staying until it's over.

◆ Have an exercise partner or go with a group.

◆ Join a walking program. Many malls now have programs where you can find like-minded (or bodied!) people who will walk with you—bad weather is no longer an excuse to avoid walking!

◆ Sign up for a race or competition.

◆ Sign up for a fitness event where you are required to raise money, such as one of the Leukemia and Lymphoma Society's prog or the Tuberous Sclerosis Complex (TSC) Association runs. These events almost always have trainers who can help motivate you and increase your fitness.

◆ Reward yourself with nonfood treats when you reach a desired goal. Then, set the next goal!

The Least You Need to Know

◆ Exercise is essential to a long health span and life span. Regular exercise will also increase your energy, vitality, and sense of well-being.

◆ Regular exercise will reduce your risk of cardiovascular disease, diabetes, arthritis, cancer, depression, and infections.

◆ All types of exercise are important for longevity—aerobic, endurance, strength training, stretching, and balance.

◆ Do at least 30 minutes of aerobic exercise most days of the week. Do strength training, stretching, and balancing at least twice weekly.

◆ Don't go overboard—excessive exercise can increase your risk of injury and infections.

Chapter 6

Ousting Obesity, Increasing Longevity

In This Chapter

- Our ever-expanding society
- Is weight *really* a product of genes?
- Never say diet
- About the National Weight Control Registry (NWCR)
- The part your brain plays
- Surgery and weight-loss drugs

Here's the simple truth: your weight has a great deal to do with the quality of your health and the length of your life. Obesity opens the door for numerous health conditions that can negatively impact your life span. Obesity is defined as having a body mass index (BMI) over 30, while overweight is a BMI between 25 and 30.

Although much research is looking at novel ways to influence your weight, well-being, and longevity through gene manipulation, for the time being we still have to address the basic laws of thermodynamics: to maintain a proper weight, you must learn to eat less and/or exercise more as you grow older. If you make good food choices, learn portion control, and stay active, you'll never need to diet. Bypass the commercialism and the diet claims and master the secrets of food—for life!

Why should you maintain a normal weight? Because maintaining a normal weight as you get older will increase your longevity. About one in eight deaths in America can be attributed to the person being overweight or obese, and some scientists predict that our current obesity epidemic will shorten life span by two to five years.

In that shortened life span, you are also more likely to suffer from chronic disease, such as heart disease, which can rob you of your health span as well. In 2001, the U.S. Surgeon General estimated that poor dietary habits and physical inactivity accounted for approximately 300,000 preventable deaths. Conversely, it's also estimated that if you're obese, just a 10 percent drop in your body weight will reduce your risk of heart disease by 20 percent. In this chapter, you'll learn how to be a thriving survivor and not an obesity statistic!

Our Culture of Affluenza

In the past, food was often a feast or famine issue. When food was available, you stuffed yourself, hoping to store up some fat and calories for the lean times that were sure to come. Many of us still have genes that adapted to that way of life and, as a result, we are very efficient at storing excess calories. Problem is, there's usually no lean time in the United States. For most of us, the food supply is always plentiful, with portion sizes growing by leaps and bounds in the past 20 years or more. Couple that with our labor-saving lifestyle, and the result is an obesity epidemic.

You've heard it before: two thirds of American adults are now overweight or obese, and obesity is also a major public health challenge for our children. The average American consumes over 3,500 calories of food per day, but the average woman needs less than 2,000 calories per day and the average man less than 3,000 per day. If you're sedentary, you need even less.

Considering that an excess of 3,500 calories adds a pound to your frame, you can see it doesn't take long to blimp out. In our culture, two very powerful forces are at work: the food industry that wants you to continue eating those excess calories (to increase profits), and the weight-loss industry that is expected to gross $60 billion in the year 2008, undoing what the food industry (and your ever-increasing consumption) has caused. Opposing forces? More likely, forces working in tandem.

The Genes in Your Jeans

Our gene pool has changed very little over the past 20 years (or 100 years, for that matter), while the incidence of overweight and obesity in the United States has sky-rocketed. What's changed is the environment. We eat, on average, about 300 more calories per day now than we did a mere 20 years ago, and we move around far less than we used to. It is true that some people do seem to be at higher genetic risk of becoming obese; they are very efficient at storing fat. If you happened to inherit those fat genes, and you love your remote and drive-thru french fries to boot, you're probably in trouble.

Newer research has shown that obese people are less genetically inclined to move, while lean people tend to just move more—they fidget, stand, pace, and tap their toes—and this nonexercise restless activity (NEAT, or nonexercise activity thermogenesis) can burn up an extra 300 calories per day. That can add up to 30 to 40 pounds of weight per year!

Longevity Facts _____

Researchers are working to identify the genes involved in weight gain and obesity, so perhaps one day we will be treating obesity with gene manipulation, rather than diet and exercise! Some scientists are also investigating the possibility that obesity may be associated with certain viral infections. If that seems like a crazy idea, doctors used to think that stress was the primary cause of stomach ulcers, and now we know that many of them are caused by bacterial infections.

The answer to avoiding excessive weight gain is self-discipline and changing some lifestyle practices. Getting up to answer the phone to parking farther away from the grocery store to standing up while you talk on the phone adds up in terms of calories burned each day.

The Great Diet Hoax

Having trouble losing weight? Most people who report the inability to lose weight, despite dieting, are grossly underestimating the number of calories they're taking in, sometimes by as much as 100 percent! They often overestimate how much exercise they're getting as well. Solution? Keep a food journal in which you write down *everything* you eat for at least several days so you can get an accurate assessment of what's going into your body. One pound of fat equals 3,500 calories, so if you want to lose 1 pound per week, you then have to reduce your daily caloric intake by 500 calories, or increase your energy expenditure by 500 calories per day, or any combination thereof. And while you're at it, slap a pedometer on your belt as well, and start measuring how many steps you're walking every day. (See Chapter 5 for more on exercise.)

Doctors' Orders

Forget about that curse word *diet*. No diet will save you. The only way to maintain a normal weight for the rest of your life is to eat healthy foods in normal portion size and exercise regularly.

If you're still not losing weight, despite your best efforts, you'll probably head to your nearest bookstore to buy the latest weight-loss diet book. There's an endless supply, and a new spate of diet books crops up every few years. There is always someone who would like to convince you that *his* or *her* diet is the one that will magically cure you, but it's just not true. There is no magical diet out there; the only diet that works is the one you stick to.

In a recent UCLA study, 31 diet studies were analyzed and compared to see how people fared in the two to five years after they lost weight on a diet. The results were that one third to two thirds of people in these studies regained their weight after they went off their diets. This is a common theme amongst dieters, who get hooked into thinking that once they get *there*, then they can relax and coast. They forget the goal is not about getting to the end zone; rather, it's about keeping to the ongoing path of well-being.

Success in keeping off the weight means paying attention to your actions day by day. If this seems hopeless at times and you sometimes feel that all you hear about is dieting failures, here's something more inspiring—the National Weight Control Registry.

The National Weight Control Registry

The National Weight Control Registry (NWCR) is a registry of people in the United States who have successfully lost at least 30 pounds and kept the weight off for at least one year. Most of the people in this group have, in fact, lost more than 60 pounds and have kept it off for five years or more.

A Little History

In the early 1990s, an ingenious nutritionist, Anne Fletcher, decided she was tired of all the pessimism in the United States about the likelihood of people losing weight *and* keeping it off. She decided to look instead at people who had been successful in the long run in their weight-loss efforts and to study them—to delve into their secrets. She called them her *masters*—people who had mastered the weight-loss game.

Not long after her first book, *Thin for Life* (see Appendix B), was published, two other researchers from Brown University and the University of Colorado, Dr. Rena Wing and Dr. James Hill, contacted Fletcher about their similar interests. Thus, in 1994, the National Weight Control Registry was born.

Anyone who has lost the requisite 30 pounds and has kept that weight off for at least a year can be a part of this database. If you are one of those folks and you would like to join, go to www.nwcr.ws. Currently, the registry is tracking over 5,000 individuals, and some of these masters have lost up to 300 pounds! They are the pioneers helping to redefine what is possible for overweight people in the United States.

Simple Secrets

What are their secrets? Their secrets are actually fairly simple. They include the following:

- They got to the point where they believed they could lose weight, even if they were overweight or obese in childhood, or even if they had made multiple attempts to lose weight and failed in the past. They finally refused to buy into the pessimism about weight-loss success.

- They have given up the words *can't* and *diet*. They have chosen to take control of their food environment. They've taken full responsibility for their weight and are determined. They also lost weight for themselves—not for their spouse, mother, or any other person. They have cultivated what psychologists call *self-efficacy*, which is one's sense of competence in a particular area.

- They don't deny themselves. They eat what they want, but in moderation. For many of them, this was their biggest breakthrough—eating what they wanted, but simply cutting back on portion sizes. And the majority do *not* feel as if they are on a diet.

- They have developed a healthy attitude about what they *should* weigh. They have given up the notion of looking like fashion models and have settled in with what feels like a healthy weight.

- They feel better having lost weight—they report improved quality of life, higher energy levels, more self-confidence, and improved physical health—and these benefits keep them committed to their healthier eating patterns.

- They have given up eating for emotional reasons. They have also given up the pity party, which led them back to unhealthy eating patterns in the past.

- The vast majority exercise at least three days per week and most of them simply engage in walking. Some do *not* exercise at all (so if the dread of exercise keeps you from tackling your weight, you can take heart).

- They give themselves permission to fail—and then they get back on track.

Healthy Practices

It's important to eat when you want to lose weight. Skipping meals only sets you up for hunger and food cravings. Eat regular meals and control your portion size. (See "Portion Psychology" later in this chapter.)

> **Words to the Wise**
>
> Whether you think you can or think you can't, either way you are right.
>
> —Henry Ford, U.S. auto manufacturer

Make each meal important. Sit down to eat. If you decide to splurge, do it with a food you *really* love—then get back on track. Eat foods that are low in fat, moderate in protein, and high in complex carbs. Drink water, instead of calorie-laden drinks. If you stock your pantry with good foods, you'll only have good choices to make!

Lifetime Weight Management

Studies of successful "losers" show that some do it just by eating smaller portions, but some find that a prescribed diet works best for them. Here's a look at some of the more popular diet plans.

The Atkins Diet

In the 1970s, nutritionists began to associate high-fat diets with heart disease and advised Americans to reduce their intake of fat. As a result, the low-fat-high-carb craze began, but alas, the incidence of obesity began to rise even further. In 1992, the Atkins Diet became immensely popular again, as the national waistline expanded. This diet gave followers free rein with high-fat foods, such as butter and bacon, but restricted all carbohydrates, including the good complex carbs that are necessary for good health. This diet often resulted in quick weight loss with improvement in lipids, but side effects were common (including bad breath and constipation). It's hard to maintain this kind of diet without getting sick of mostly fatty foods; in addition, nutrition experts worried about the long-term impact of high–animal fat diets on cardiovascular health.

The Ornish Plan

Dean Ornish, M.D., was one of the first researchers to show that heart disease could be reversed with a strict diet. The Ornish Plan consisted of severe fat restriction (less than 5 percent of calories from fat each day), lots of complex carbs, exercise, meditation, and weekly support groups. Although his plan did help many of his patients reverse heart disease and restore health, its restrictive nature made it difficult for many people to maintain.

The Mediterranean Diet

In the 1950s, nutrition researchers began what was called the Seven Countries Study, the first major study to examine the relationship between diet and heart disease. This study looked at the dietary patterns in seven Mediterranean countries, including Greece and southern Italy—areas of the world where people enjoyed long lives generally free of heart disease and some cancers. Diets in this part of the world consisted mainly of plant-based foods, including fruits, veggies, beans, unrefined grains, nuts, seeds, and olive oil. Animal foods, such as dairy products, meat, and poultry, were eaten sparingly.

Thus the Mediterranean diet was born; this diet is now advocated by many as one of the healthiest and most longevity-advancing diets in the world. However, it can be easy to pack on the calories if you load up on olive oil. Stick with the plant-based focus and you should lose weight *and* live longer!

The Volumetrics Plan

Barbara Rolls, Ph.D., a well-known nutrition researcher at Penn State University, introduced the concept of *energy density* into the weight-loss equation, and her weight-loss advice is highly regarded by many in the field. Energy density is the number of calories in a gram of food. A food with a high energy density (such as a candy bar) has a lot of calories per gram. Fat is the biggest contributor to the energy density of a food, while a food high in water content, such as watermelon, has a much lower energy density.

Dr. Rolls found that people tend to stop eating when they get full, and fullness or satiety is determined in part by the *volume* or weight of food eaten, not by the energy density. She also found that we all tend to eat the same weight of food day after day, so by choosing foods high in volume and low in energy density, we will get full quickly on fewer calories. For example, 2 cups of grapes containing 100 calories will fill you up and satisfy your hunger far more than ¼ cup of raisins, which also has 100 calories. If you choose the raisins over the grapes, you will get hungry again more quickly and take in more calories overall. Lowering the energy density of your meals will result in an overall lower calorie intake.

Longevity Facts

Foods with a very low calorie density (less than 0.60) include lettuce, tomato, watermelon, broccoli, vegetable soup, and oranges. Foods with a low density (0.60–1.5) include rice, oatmeal, grapes, baked potato with skin, and black beans. Foods with a medium density (1.6–3.9) include bread, cheese pizza, raisins, hard pretzels, and lean ground meat. Foods with a high density (4.0 and over) include butter, bacon, cheddar cheese, and almonds.

Foods with high water content, such as fruits and veggies, are high in volume and low in calories. Choosing to eat these *first* in a meal might fill you, before you want that helping of french fries. Drinking water before a meal, an often-advised practice to reduce hunger, doesn't work as well. A glass of water empties out of the stomach fairly quickly and doesn't always reduce hunger. However, having a cup of low-fat soup before a meal does tend to fill you up and reduce the overall calories that you will take in. Start with a cup of soup before every dinner and you are on your way to weight loss!

Doctors' Orders

If you're trying to reduce your caloric intake, diet beverages are certainly better than drinking full-calorie fluids, but some health experts feel that the continued consumption of diet foods conditions us to crave more sweet stuff, including the nondiet variety. Try blending soda water with a little orange juice for a healthier beverage that gives you some nutrients to boot.

Fiber and protein also increase satiety (even more than fat). Adding these to each meal will also help reduce overall food intake, along with food cravings. With a little practice, you can switch around the foods you choose and trick your stomach into wanting less. The Volumetrics diet is probably one of the most effective ways to lose weight. Of course, you will still need to pay attention to what goes into your mouth, including your portion sizes, but when you reduce both portion size and calorie density, you may reduce your caloric intake by up to 800 calories per day and not feel deprived—how easy could it get? And of course, don't forget to exercise!

An Overall Plan

What's the average consumer to do in this morass of diet books, weight-loss products, and other hype out there? If it sounds too good to be true, it's almost guaranteed that it is. Lean toward a Mediterranean-type diet for overall good health; be sure to get healthy protein, fiber, and fat at every meal to enhance your satiety; and choose high-volume, low-calorie (low energy density) foods, which will fill you up and tell your brain satiety meter that it's time to close up the kitchen.

Engaging Your Brain

Your brain has a lot to do with your appetite, food intake, and weight. Learning how to harness your brain for health, weight control, and increased life span is important to your success in these areas.

Stress tends to drive up your appetite, especially for high-fat, high-calorie foods. Finding ways to reduce the perception of stress in your life is paramount in weight loss. In a similar vein, unresolved emotional issues from the past, including any history of abuse, can sabotage your weight-loss efforts. It's estimated that about 8 percent of obese people in the United States were abused in some way in childhood. Understand the connection between your use of food and your psychological and emotional health.

Sleep Deprivation

Many Americans do not get enough sleep. Sleep deprivation leads to impaired ability to handle blood sugar and also leads to increased insulin levels—both risk factors for diabetes.

Sleep deprivation also leads to changes in the hormones that control appetite. Leptin, a hormone that suppresses appetite by signaling the brain that we're full, drops during sleep deprivation. The hormone ghrelin, which stimulates appetite, goes up, leading to increased food intake, weight gain, and obesity.

Portion Psychology

Many people who are successful at weight loss learn to control their portions. One way to do this is to use smaller plates and bowls. Studies have shown that you will put less food on them and eat fewer calories overall. If you enjoy eating out, consider splitting your entrée in two when it arrives at the table and taking the leftovers home. Likewise, it's probably best to stay away from buffet lines and all-you-can-eat specials. An endless supply and variety of foods stimulates the appetite and lulls you into eating, even if you're not hungry anymore.

Happy Frontal Lobes

Recent fascinating research suggests that the frontal lobes of the brain, especially on the right side, have an impact on eating behavior. Reduced function or damage to this part of the brain may lead to overeating, as well as reduced physical activity. Conversely, exercise can increase the volume and function of the brain in the right frontal lobe, which, in turn, might lead to reduced food craving. Perhaps this is one of the mechanisms whereby exercise helps people to reduce their weight and keep it off.

Hormones and neurotransmitters in the brain that seem to affect appetite, such as insulin, cortisol, leptin, and ghrelin, all seem to affect this part of the brain as well. Stay tuned as this type of brain research evolves, but in the meantime, don't forget to exercise!

Bariatric Surgery

If your BMI is over 40 (severe or morbid obesity) or your BMI is over 35 and you have health problems aggravated by obesity, including heart disease and diabetes, your doctor may refer you for bariatric surgery. Bariatric surgery refers to operations performed to promote weight loss. Bariatric surgeries generally fall into three categories: gastric banding, gastric bypass surgery, and an even more invasive bypass surgery known as the duodenal switch. All of these procedures tend to produce a fair amount of weight loss in the first few years after they are done; by 10 years out, however, the only ones that seem to produce significant persistent weight loss are the bypass procedures.

Longevity Facts _____

The following are the recommended classifications for BMI adopted by the National Institutes of Health (NIH) and World Health Organization (WHO). These are endorsed by most expert groups:

◆ Underweight: BMI is less than 18.5 kg/m².

◆ Normal weight: BMI is equal to or greater than 18.5 to 24.9 kg/m².

◆ Overweight: BMI is equal to or greater than 25.0 to 29.9 kg/m².

◆ Class I obesity: BMI equals 30.0 to 34.9 kg/m².

◆ Class II obesity: BMI equals 35.0 to 39.9 kg/m².

◆ Class III obesity: BMI is equal to or greater than 40 kg/m². This type of obesity is also referred to as severe, extreme, or morbid obesity.

Gastric Banding

This procedure involves placing a silicone band around the upper part of the stomach and tightening it to create a small upper stomach through which food must pass. The band is generally inflatable; inflating it more tightens the band, reduces the size of the stomach pouch, and leads to more weight loss. Forty to 60 percent of excess weight is initially lost after this procedure. As with the vertical band, long-term success is much lower.

Gastric Bypass

The procedure most commonly done now is called the Roux-en-Y procedure. This operation reduces the stomach to a small pouch. Part of the small intestine is then bypassed, and the remaining small intestine is attached to the stomach pouch. Patients lose up to 80 percent of their excess weight with this type of procedure. Complications can include surgical risks, such as bleeding and infections. Significant nutrient deficiencies may also develop, and patients must take vitamin and mineral supplements for the rest of their lives.

Duodenal Switch

This surgery is more drastic than the previous two; it switches a portion of the duodenum and stomach and bypasses a large part of the intestines so that less food is absorbed. It also leads to more nutrient depletion than the standard bypass and is usually reserved for patients with a BMI greater than 50.

Bariatric Surgery and Longevity

The weight loss that people achieve from these surgeries does reduce risks of diabetes, high blood pressure, and high cholesterol. What has been unclear is whether or not *longevity* is increased as well. However, a recent study of over 4,000 obese people from Sweden suggests that it is. These researchers compared obese people who had one of the above three surgeries with people who received conventional treatment. At the end of an average of 11 years of follow-up, those who had the surgery had about a 30 percent reduction in mortality.

> **Words to the Wise**
>
> If you are considering one of these procedures, be sure to look for an accredited surgeon who is a member of the American Society of Bariatric Surgeons. The procedure should be done in a hospital that has been designated by this organization as a "Center of Excellence."

There are many other benefits as well. Multiple medical problems associated with obesity tend to resolve with persistent weight loss from these surgeries, including heart disease, diabetes, high blood pressure, high cholesterol, sleep apnea, depression, asthma, migraine headaches, and arthritis.

Weight-Loss Drugs

Weight-loss drugs work in various ways; all of them require a prescription, except as indicated:

- Stimulants, such as amphetamines and fen-phen, work by suppressing appetite but are associated with potentially serious side effects.

- Meridia suppresses appetite, can increase blood pressure, and may also be associated with other serious problems.

- Orlistat (also sold as nonprescription alli) blocks fat absorption in the gut. Side effects include greasy diarrhea and fat-soluble vitamin deficiencies.

- Topamax, a drug developed for seizures, reduces appetite and produces some weight loss. It can also cause fatigue and other side effects.

- Wellbutrin, a drug used for depression, may result in reduced appetite and weight loss in some patients, although it is not FDA-approved for this purpose.

- Accomplia is a new prescription drug that reduces appetite by blocking cannabinoid receptors in the brain. It has significant side effects, including anxiety and depression.

◆ Over-the-counter supplements, such as ma huang, bitter orange, and country mallow, act as stimulants which may suppress appetite. They have become popular since the FDA pulled ephedra from the shelves in 2004, but there is no good data that they produce any significant weight loss.

None of these meds are approved by the FDA for long-term use for weight loss. There is also no good data suggesting they do anything to increase longevity. They are always meant to be used in conjunction with a weight-loss program that includes healthy diet, regular exercise, and medical supervision.

In the future, there will probably be new gene and hormone therapies available that will suppress appetite, increase metabolism and energy expenditure, and help us to maintain a healthy weight. In the meantime, avoid the temptation of over-portioned and nutrient-dense restaurant foods and beverages, eat high-volume foods, follow a Mediterranean-type diet, and keep your walking shoes on!

The Least You Need to Know

◆ Longevity is enhanced when you maintain a healthy weight throughout your life. Obesity increases your risk of chronic disease and shortens your life span.

◆ You must consciously choose to be responsible for your weight.

◆ If you eat healthy whole foods low in energy density, now and forever, you will successfully maintain your weight.

◆ Exercise not only burns calories and increases your muscle mass but may also influence your brain health, which in turn affects your appetite and desire to eat.

◆ Getting enough sleep, reducing stress, and healing any unresolved emotional baggage will increase your success at weight loss.

◆ Weight-loss surgery is generally successful in helping very obese people lose weight. It also seems to improve their longevity. Weight-loss drugs, on the other hand, are generally much less effective.

Chapter 7

Supplements

In This Chapter

- ◆ Your health and supplements
- ◆ Vitamins: learning your ABCs
- ◆ Rock-solid information about necessary minerals
- ◆ Herbs, spices, and other botanicals
- ◆ How to be an educated consumer

Vitamins, minerals, and other nutrients found in food are the building blocks of life. You know you get them from what you eat, so do you really need to take them in the form of supplements? Will they really make a difference in your health or your longevity? In this chapter, you'll learn which products can truly be beneficial and which to leave alone.

Necessity or Hype?

Supplements are everywhere; you'll find them on pharmacy shelves, in supermarkets and health-food stores, and on the Internet. Although manufacturers can't make specific health claims for their products, they can make structure and function claims designed to lead you to believe supplements will cure everything from diarrhea to dementia.

Humans have gotten by without supplements for thousands of years. Primitive peoples ate the plants and animals available in their local environments. Although their longevity was shortened by traumas and infectious diseases that no longer affect us, these peoples were largely free of the chronic diseases that now shorten our lives. Many of us have bought into the supplement culture and have come to rely on supplement pills to provide us with our essential nutrients. In so doing, we miss out on the phytochemicals in food that are as yet unavailable in pill form. There is still no substitute for that bowl of spectacular salad.

def•i•ni•tion

Supplements fall into the following categories: vitamins, minerals, herbs and spices, other botanicals or plant chemicals, and mixtures of these categories (such as multivitamin/mineral pills).

Deficiencies in Our Midst

Focus first on your food. Many Americans of all ages are short on important nutrients in their diets, including B vitamins, vitamin D, calcium, and iron. Deficiencies in some of these can have serious consequences, such as birth defects. Other subtle deficiencies probably exist that contribute more quietly to chronic diseases, including cancer and Alzheimer's disease. While some supplements are worth taking, especially for those days when you don't get in all of those fruits and veggies, others are not. A good time to talk to your doctor about supplements is at your yearly visit.

A Multi-Billion-Dollar Industry

Supplements are *big* business. In 2004, more than 50 percent of Americans took dietary supplements, spending more than $20 billion on these products. Studies have shown that many people will continue to take a particular supplement even if studies suggest that that supplement does not work.

Vitamins

Vitamins are natural compounds found in plant and animal food; they are only needed in relatively small quantities but are essential for life. Until the twentieth century, people obtained their vitamins and other nutrients from natural sources only. The primary source was food. Consumption of vitamins and minerals in pill form is a relatively recent phenomenon. Vitamins are broadly classified into water soluble and fat soluble:

◆ *Water soluble* vitamins include vitamin C and the nine B vitamins. While some water soluble vitamins can cause side effects if taken in large quantities, excesses in the blood are generally excreted in the urine without problems.

◆ *Fat soluble* vitamins are A, D, E, and K. The carotenoids, which are also fat soluble, are essential ingredients to good health. Many carotenoids serve as precursors to vitamin A. Fat soluble vitamins can cause problems if taken in large quantities. Because these vitamins are soluble in fat, they are stored in human fatty tissue, including the brain, and can cause toxicity if taken in excess, especially vitamins A and D.

Antioxidants

Normal metabolic processes, including the breakdown and metabolism of foods, produce reactive oxygen molecules, called free radicals. Left unchecked, these free radicals can damage other cells, leading to cell breakdown and possibly even cancerous transformation. Antioxidants are substances, usually found in foods, that neutralize these free radicals, thus restoring the body's chemical balance.

Nature usually creates just enough antioxidants in our food to balance the oxidants produced in our bodies. Major changes in our food supply, especially the enormous shift away from omega-3 fats toward the more inflammatory omega-6 fats, along with the lack of fruits and veggies in our diets, has tipped the scale toward an inflammatory state for many of us. Additionally, environmental pollutants, such as smoke and ionizing radiation, add their share of free radicals. Many experts now feel that free radical damage to our cells and DNA plays a major role in accelerating the aging process.

The question that logically follows is, "Will taking antioxidants in pill form keep you healthy and stave off aging and chronic disease?" Studies in this area so far have been disappointing. Nature remains the best source of antioxidants.

The one exception here might be taking supplements to reduce your risk of macular degeneration, the most common cause of age-related reversible blindness in the United States. One important study that looked at the impact of several supplements on disease progression in people with moderate macular degeneration found that a daily combination of supplemental zinc, copper, vitamin E, and beta-carotene taken together seemed to reduce the risk of progression of macular degeneration by 25 percent in people who already had moderate disease. As always, talk to your doctor before starting these supplements.

In the vitamin category, nature's best antioxidants include vitamins C and E, as well as the carotenes. The minerals selenium and zinc are also considered antioxidants, as are many other plant chemicals, such as the polyphenols. The human body also manufactures its own supply of antioxidants, especially glutathione and super oxide dismutase; these are not available in pill form.

Getting at least some of your antioxidants in pill form may provide you with some insurance. Most of us can get what we need in a multivitamin. Taking an individual supplement or vitamin alone often doesn't work; antioxidants probably need each other to work effectively.

Vitamins C and E and selenium are available in supplement form. Beta-carotene should be obtained from food, especially if you smoke. One medium-size carrot will give you most of your daily requirement of beta-carotene. The other carotenes, such as lutein and zeaxanthin, can be taken in pill form. On a cautionary note, studies have shown that smokers who take beta-carotene supplements have a *higher* risk of lung cancer than those who avoid this supplement.

Vitamin C

Vitamin C is *the* proto-typical antioxidant, protecting the body's tissues from the harmful effects of inflammation. It is also needed for the healthy operation of many enzymes in the body, as well as for the synthesis of collagen. Vitamin C is found primarily in fruits and vegetables, and some is also available in animal food, especially liver. Unlike many other mammals, humans cannot synthesize their own vitamin C and must obtain it from food. Because mammals that *do* make vitamin C can produce thousands of milligrams per day, advocates of large supplements of vitamin C feel that humans should probably get similar intakes or at least considerably more than current recommended amounts.

Doctors' Orders

Nobel Prize Laureate Linus Pauling was one of the leading proponents of large intakes of vitamin C, sometimes taking over 10 g per day himself. Advocates claim that large doses can help prevent or treat many diseases and conditions, including viral infections (including HIV and bird flu) and heart disease. Vitamin C is also currently being studied in high intravenous doses for use in terminally ill cancer patients. Most of the data supporting large doses, however, has been controversial.

Vitamin C is safe in reasonable doses. It is estimated that tissues are saturated at a dose of about 250 *mg*, though the recommended daily dose is 90 mg per day for men and 75 for women. Smokers should add an additional 35 mg per day because their metabolic

def•i•ni•tion

Understanding dosage definitions is important: **mg** stands for milligram; **mcgm** stands for microgram.

turnover of vitamin C is more rapid, as is their rate of oxidative stress. At least half of this can be obtained by eating 5 to 10 servings of fruits and veggies every day. For some people, high doses of vitamin C can cause stomach upset, diarrhea, flushing, and headache. Also, vitamin C increases the absorption of iron. For someone with an undiagnosed case of iron storage disease (hemochromatosis), excess vitamin C can worsen iron overload, increasing the risk of liver and other organ failure.

B Vitamins

B vitamins are also water soluble and are found in both plant and animal food. They have a broad array of functions. Many come packaged together in foods and often need each other to work optimally. That's why almost every multivitamin on the shelf contains a complex of B vitamins and not just one or two alone. Taking just one or two in supplement form and leaving the others out can lead to imbalance, so take them in *B-complex* form. One exception to this is B_{12}. Many of us do need this one alone in larger amounts as we get older. If you take folate alone, you may mask a vitamin B_{12} deficiency, so take your B-complex supplement!

Because so many foods are fortified with B vitamins, it's unlikely you'll need all of the other B vitamins in large amounts, or as individual supplements. Look for a multivitamin containing the daily value of the other B vitamins, including B_1 (thiamin), B_2 (riboflavin), B_3 (niacin), B_5 (pantothenic acid), B_6 (pyridoxine), and biotin. Three of the B vitamins are especially important—folate, B_6, and B_{12}:

◆ Folate is extremely important for general health. Deficiency leads to birth defects, including spina bifida. For older folks, adequate folate may protect from heart disease and cancer, especially pancreatic cancer and possibly colon and esophageal cancer. Folate is mainly found in leafy green veggies. Take as a B-complex, multivitamin, or B-complex tab. Recommended dose: 400 to 800 *mcgm* per day.

◆ Vitamin B_6 is important for heart health and also needed for the manufacture of serotonin, an important chemical in the brain that helps prevent depression. B_6 is found in fortified cereals, meats, nuts, and beans. Take it in a multivitamin. Recommended dose: 1.3 to 1.7 mg per day.

◆ Vitamin B$_{12}$ has many functions, including keeping the brain, heart, arteries, and nervous system healthy. It also nourishes red blood cells. It's found only in animal foods, such as meat, poultry, fish, and dairy. Vegetarians and vegans will need to take this in supplement form. As we age, many of us absorb B$_{12}$ much less efficiently from food, so taking it in supplement form is helpful. Only small amounts are generally needed. The *silver* multivitamins, designed for adults over 50, contain the higher amounts needed for this age group. Recommended dose: 2.5 to 25 mcgm per day.

Vitamin A and the Carotenes

Vitamin A comes in two forms: pre-formed vitamin A (retinol), which is found only in animal foods, and pro–vitamin A carotenes—such as beta-carotene—found in fruits and veggies. Vitamin A is important for healthy vision, helps regulate cell growth, and is essential for maintaining a healthy immune system as we get older. Some data suggests that inadequate intake can increase the risk of cancer.

Pre-formed vitamin A can be toxic when you take more than you need. For example, too much increases your risk of osteoporosis; for this reason, the government recently reduced the recommended amount of daily vitamin A to 2,310 International Units (IU) for women or 2,565 for men.

Pro–vitamin A compounds, or carotenes, are also fat soluble but are not associated with toxicity, as long as they are obtained from food. Beta-carotene supplements, however, have been associated with an increased risk of cancer, especially lung cancer in smokers. It's easy to get plenty of carotenes from your food supply, as long as you eat lots of fruits and veggies. In general, it's not necessary to take carotene supplements, although supplemental beta-carotene has been used to slow the progression of macular degeneration. Talk with your doctor before you take these supplements.

Vitamin D

Vitamin D is perhaps best known for its role in bone health and in osteoporosis prevention but also seems to be important for the optimal health and longevity of *most* of our tissues. Research suggests that adequate vitamin D may help prevent:

◆ Osteoporosis

◆ Muscle weakness, leading to increased risk of falls, especially in the elderly

♦ Cancer, especially colon cancer and perhaps breast cancer as well

♦ Type 2 (adult-onset) diabetes

♦ Infections

♦ Autoimmune diseases, including type 1 diabetes, multiple sclerosis, and rheumatoid arthritis

♦ Osteoarthritis progression

♦ Periodontal (gum) disease and tooth loss

Some studies suggest we are deficient in vitamin D, which is manufactured in our skin when we are exposed to the sun. The skin's ability to do this declines as we age, if we live in more northern latitudes, and also during nonsummer months. Someone living near the equator could manufacture thousands of units of vitamin D per day. Unfortunately, most of us spend our days inside, and when outside, slather on sunscreen, which inhibits our body's ability to make vitamin D.

Consider getting your vitamin D blood level checked; an ideal level is probably at least 50 nanomoles per liter; taking 1,000 units per day total (from food and supplements together) should be enough. Maximum recommended intake is 2,000 units per day, though medical studies currently underway are testing the efficacy and safety of higher doses. Higher doses of D *may* increase your risk of kidney stones, so be sure to talk to your doctor first if you have a personal or family history of this. When purchasing a supplement, look for vitamin D_3, or "cholecalciferol," which is more potent than other forms of D.

Vitamin E

Recent studies suggest that vitamin E doesn't seem to prevent heart disease and cancer as was first thought. On the other hand, populations of people who get more vitamin E in their diets *do* seem to have less heart disease and cancer. Why the discrepancy? Vitamin E may need other antioxidants with it in order to do its job optimally. Also, some studies may not have been long enough to show the potential benefit of vitamin E. Studies in Alzheimer's patients and in people with macular degeneration have shown that vitamin E may slow the progression of those diseases somewhat. More studies are underway. In the meantime, take a multivitamin that has at least some E in it; if you take an additional supplement, keep it under 400 mg per day. Vitamin E can thin the blood a bit, so talk to your doctor first if you are already taking blood thinners.

Vitamin K

Vitamin K is the last of the fat soluble vitamins and is best known for its role in helping the blood to clot. Recent research has shown that this vitamin also plays an important role in bone health, for example, in preventing osteoporosis. Women with low vitamin K intakes are twice as likely to break a hip as women with adequate intakes. Vitamin K is most plentiful in fruits and veggies, especially the dark green ones. The government recommends that you look for a multivitamin containing vitamin K. One cautionary note: vitamin K interferes with blood thinners, so talk to your doctor first if you are taking them. The recommended daily intake is 150 to 250 mcgm per day from food and/or your multivitamin.

Minerals

Minerals are essential components of blood, organs, and other tissues. Minerals also drive the body's enzyme systems, allowing biochemical reactions to take place. All are necessary, and some are really worth taking as supplements.

Although body tissues may seem soft, your body contains lots of minerals. In fact, someone once described the human body as a rock—filled with calcium, magnesium, crystals, and many other minerals you'd expect to find in your average boulder!

Doctors' Orders

Any mineral taken in excess can be toxic. In particular, watch out for selenium, which can become toxic in high doses. Also, taking too much zinc can reduce your absorption of copper and lead to a deficiency here. Again, check with your doctor before starting supplements.

Calcium

Many Americans do not get enough calcium, especially teenagers, pregnant women, and post-menopausal women. The health concern most of us hear about is osteoporosis, or frail, easily fractured bones. Bone health is established in childhood and young adulthood by eating a healthy diet that includes lots of calcium, fruits, veggies, and also includes getting plenty of exercise. Skimp here and your risk of osteoporosis increases as you age. As you'll see in Chapter 15, breaking a bone—especially your hip in later years—is a sure way to reduce your longevity.

The average amount recommended for adults is 1,200 mg per day and is best obtained through diet. If you take it as a supplement, it's best absorbed if you divide it up and take 400 to 500 mg three times a day with meals.

Calcium carbonate is the most widely used calcium supplement (TUMS are often used for this purpose). If this causes any stomach upset for you, or if you have reduced stomach acid for any reason (especially if you're one of those folks taking meds for chronic acid, such as Prilosec or Zantac), then try calcium citrate instead. You'll have to take more of these pills to get the same amount of calcium in calcium carbonate, however, so read those labels!

Doctors' Orders

Avoid bone meal as a calcium supplement; it may be contaminated with lead and other harmful substances.

Iron

Many people are deficient in iron, especially vegetarians and those with poor diets. Iron is found mainly in animal foods, such as red meat, and also in some vegetable foods, though it is less well-absorbed from vegetables than meat. Most of the iron in your body is carried in your red blood cells. Iron deficiency leads to anemia, fatigue, and weakness. Because only tiny amounts of iron are lost from the body in the stool, if you are an older adult found to have iron deficiency, you are considered to be losing blood from your GI tract until proven otherwise. Likely culprits here are gastritis, diverticulitis, colon polyps, or colon cancer. If you have iron deficiency, get a GI tract workup. The recommended amount is 18 mg per day for menstruating women, and 8 mg per day for men and for women who are no longer menstruating; pregnant women need a bit more.

Potassium

Potassium is found primarily in fruits and veggies in the form of potassium citrate. Many of us think of potassium as a supplemental medicine (usually potassium chloride) that we take with a diuretic (water pill). Potassium is a much bigger player than that, however. Potassium deficiency probably aggravates high blood pressure and increases your risk of osteoporosis. The recommended dose is 4,700 mg per day, preferably from your food and not taken as a supplement pill.

Magnesium

Studies suggest that magnesium, especially from foods, can lower blood pressure, protect bones, and may even reduce your risk of diabetes. The recommended dose is 400 to 500 mg per day. The best food sources for magnesium are vegetables, legumes, seafood, nuts, and dairy.

Selenium

Selenium is both a mineral and an antioxidant. It is important for the health of your immune system and thyroid gland. A recent study has suggested that selenium can protect from cancer, including prostate cancer and skin cancer. However, selenium is toxic if overconsumed. The amount in our diets is largely determined by the selenium content of the soil in which the food was grown, and this varies widely across the country. The recommended intake is about 55 mcgm per day, which can usually be obtained in a multivitamin.

Zinc and Copper

Zinc is important for a healthy immune system and may also function as an antioxidant. It is plentiful in animal foods, including dairy products. Many folks take zinc lozenges for colds, but taking high doses for long periods of time suppresses your immune system and leads to copper and iron deficiency, which may cause anemia; it may even lower your HDL (good) cholesterol. Don't exceed 15 to 20 mg per day from supplements.

Like zinc, copper also seems to function as an antioxidant and is important for blood cell production, as well as bone and joint health. The recommended dose is about 900 mcgm per day. Many Americans may not get enough copper in their diets. The best dietary sources are legumes, nuts, and meat. Zinc, iron, and vitamin C can all interfere with copper absorption or utilization.

Supplemental zinc and copper have been used in combination with beta-carotene and vitamin E to slow the progression of macular degeneration. Speak with your doctor before beginning these supplements.

Chromium

Many supplement manufacturers have claimed chromium can reduce blood sugar and blood lipids and also help people lose weight, but this only seems to hold true for people who are chromium deficient to begin with (and this is rare). Meats and whole grains are great sources. The current recommended dose is 20 to 30 mcgm per day.

Sodium

Americans eat *way too much* sodium. Too much sodium = high blood pressure, stroke, and heart disease = a shortened life span! Only about 10 percent of our salt intake comes from the salt shaker; the vast majority comes from restaurant and/or processed foods. Read those food labels and ask your restaurant to provide you with the sodium content of their foods. If you can, try to limit your intake to 1,500 mg per day, especially if you have hypertension or heart disease.

The Herb and Spice Garden

Herbs and spices have been used medicinally in many cultures for thousands of years. They are now widely used in the West as well. Will they increase your longevity? Some may, and many are useful for ailments that become more common as we age. In that capacity, they can reduce symptoms and improve quality of life.

Keep in mind that herbs contain chemicals, much as prescription drugs do. They can be beneficial but can also be toxic when taken inappropriately. Many of them also interact with prescription medications and with each other. Consult with your doctor before taking any herbal supplements.

Turmeric

Animal studies of curcumin, the active chemical in the herb turmeric, show possible benefit in reducing the incidence and spread of cancer and brain disease, including Alzheimer's. Human studies are underway. In the meantime, reasonable doses are probably safe, especially if you are at risk of brain disease. Stick with 2,000 mg per day or less. This herb can interfere with the metabolism of prescription meds, so talk to your doctor before starting.

Cinnamon

A small but promising study done at the USDA several years ago showed that as little as ½ teaspoon of grocery store cinnamon per day lowered blood sugar, cholesterol, and triglycerides. However, subsequent studies have failed to show such a great benefit (further investigation is being done). Consider taking it in supplement form: cinnamon supplements are made by extracting the active ingredients from the spice, and this process also removes potential harmful substances, including coumarins that can thin your blood. The dose used in studies has been 1 to 6 g per day (1 teaspoon contains 4.75 g of cinnamon).

Garlic

Garlic has been used medicinally for thousands of years. Will it help you to live longer? It has been shown to have numerous health benefits, especially when it comes to your heart. Garlic seems to reduce stiffness in the arteries and may also reduce heart disease and high blood pressure; all of these benefits can help you live longer.

Black Cohosh

Black cohosh, an herb traditionally used by Native Americans for female disorders, is used most often in the West to reduce vasomotor symptoms during menopause, though data has not been conclusive. It is imported from Germany by Glaxo under the name Remifemin. The dose is 20 mg twice daily for six months. The safety of long-term use is not known; in addition, some studies have suggested liver damage with black cohosh, though this was probably caused by impurities in the supplement and not by the herb itself. If you're considering black cohosh, stick with Remifemin, which is a standardized product.

Other Botanicals

Many plant chemicals in our foods have yet to be identified. As you can guess, nature put many of them there for a reason—and it usually has to do with good health and long life. While some of these chemicals have been isolated and are now available in pill form, focus on getting yours from fruits, vegetables, and other plant foods.

Polyphenols

Polyphenols are chemicals found in plant foods and so named because they have the basic structure of phenol carbon rings. Most polyphenols act as antioxidants and cancer-fighting chemicals in the body. How they do that is not completely clear; they may induce enzymes that are health-enhancing or they may have direct effects themselves.

Polyphenols are abundant in berries, tea, red grapes/wine, extra-virgin olive oil, dark chocolate, walnuts, fruits, veggies, and other plant foods. They are generally broken down into three broad groups: flavonoids, tannins, and lignans.

One especially intriguing flavonoid is resveratrol, which is found in many plant foods and is especially abundant in the skin of grapes. It is an antioxidant produced when plants are grown in stressful conditions, and it seems to prolong life; at least it seems to do this in yeast cells growing in the laboratory. This may, in part, explain the longevity of people who drink red wine on a regular basis, such as people living in the Mediterranean.

Phytoestrogens (plant hormones) are another frequently used plant substance; they are found in the polyphenol group known as lignans. They may relieve menopausal symptoms in some women, although the placebo effect is very high. Soy foods do help some women, however, and soy is a great source of plant protein. Long-term safety of phytoestrogen pills is unknown, especially if you are at risk for breast cancer.

Fish Oil

Fish oils containing the essential oils EPA and DHA seem to prevent heart attacks, slow the progression of heart disease, and also reduce the risk of sudden death from heart disease, thus enhancing longevity. They are powerful anti-inflammatories and may also reduce the risk of asthma and numerous other conditions associated with inflammation. The American Heart Association now recommends that people with heart disease or those at risk for heart disease consume fish or fish oil tablets on a regular basis. Take roughly 1,000 mg per day of EPA/DHA combined.

Alpha-Lipoic Acid

Alpha-lipoic acid (ALA) is a powerful antioxidant that may also help relieve neuropathy, or irritation of the nerves, especially in diabetics. It also enhances the activity of insulin. The effective dose is 600 mg twice daily.

Red Yeast Rice

Red yeast rice is rice that has been fermented with the yeast *Monascus purpureus*. This fermentation process produces a chemical identical to the drug Mevacor (lovastatin), a cholesterol-lowering statin drug. Statins have been shown to enhance longevity in people with vascular disease and diabetes. People taking these products need to have their liver function tests monitored, as both red yeast rice and statins can irritate the liver. There have been some recent FDA concerns regarding the use of red yeast rice, so talk to your doctor before taking this product.

Acetyl-L-Carnitine

Acetyl-L-carnitine (ALC) is an amino acid that helps increase acetylcholine in the brain and has been studied for use in Alzheimer's. (Alzheimer's patients' brains are deficient in this.) The dose used in studies has been 1,500 to 4,000 mg per day in divided doses. It seems to be safe but can cause some stomach upset. ALC also shows promise for patients with neuropathy, including diabetic neuropathy. If you take blood thinners, especially Coumadin, talk to your doctor before taking ALC, as it can increase Coumadin's effects.

CoEnzyme Q-10

Co Q-10 is an antioxidant involved in cell energy metabolism. It has been used for many medical conditions, including congestive heart failure (100 mg per day), high blood pressure (60 mg twice per day), and migraine headaches (100 mg three times per day). It may also help relieve the muscle pain that many people experience when they take statin drugs for high cholesterol. In high doses, it may also slow the rate of decline for people with early Parkinson's disease.

Choosing Products Wisely

The FDA does not regulate vitamins, minerals, herbs, amino acids, and other supplements. Educating yourself as to their safety and efficacy is essential to your health and longevity. Here are a few tips:

- ◆ Look for products that have the designation "USP" (US Pharmacopoeia), "NF" (National Formulary), or "GMP" (Good Manufacturing Practices). This suggests they have undergone some evaluation of their purity. (Manufacturers submit to this on a voluntary basis.) *Consumer Reports* has also begun rating supplement products.

- Buy brand-name products from reputable companies, such as Whitehall Robbins, Centrum Herbals, and Bayer One-A-Day Herbals.

- Search for reliable information on medical websites. WebMD (www.webmd.com) is a good source, as are most of the websites at academic universities. The Office of Dietary Supplements at the National Institutes of Health (NIH) is excellent; its website is http://dietary-supplements.info. nih.gov.

> **Words to the Wise**
>
> If you use supplements regularly, consider subscribing to www. consumerlab.com ($29.95/year). This is an independent testing lab, providing information about the purity and quality of a wide number of brand-name products on the market.

The Least You Need to Know

- Supplements include vitamins, minerals, herbs and spices, other botanicals or plant chemicals, and mixtures of these categories.

- Most of the nutrients we need can be obtained from our diets, as long as we maximize our intake of fruits, vegetables, whole grains, and healthy oils.

- If you are unable to eat a balanced diet for any reason, then consider taking a daily multivitamin or mineral supplement for insurance.

- Some supplements are beneficial; others are potentially harmful. Always consult with your physician before beginning any supplement regimen.

- If you take supplements on a regular basis, educate yourself on the quality, purity, and effectiveness of what you take.

Chapter 8

Creating Restorative Sleep

In This Chapter

- ◆ Why sleep is so important
- ◆ REM and non-REM sleep
- ◆ The effects of sleep deprivation
- ◆ Medical conditions and other factors that affect your sleep
- ◆ Medications and alternative sleep therapies

Developing great sleep habits is one of the best things you can do for your health and your longevity. People who don't sleep enough, don't sleep regularly, or don't sleep soundly are at increased risk of chronic disease and a shortened life span. To live longer and better, learn to sleep well!

The Importance of a Good Night's Sleep

Ah, a good night's sleep—something many of us find elusive as we get older. For many Americans, sleep deprivation is a lifestyle choice and not an inevitable part of aging. Sleep patterns and needs tend to change as you age, but if you learn to flow with this change, you can reclaim your right to a restful night. Want to enhance your longevity? Then don't scrimp on sleep!

Snuggle down in those covers and get your zzzz's. Having trouble with your sleep? Whether you fall asleep quickly and then wake up or you find you can't drift off at all, there is help!

Around the turn of the last century, the average person got about nine hours of sleep. These days, many of us are lucky to get five or six. In our hectic lives, we tend to think of sleep as a luxury, not something that's essential to our survival. As a consequence, we use time we should be sleeping as "found time" in which we attempt to squeeze in a few more tasks and do a little more work. We're literally starving our body of an essential requirement: sleep.

Longevity Facts

The now famous Alameda County Study conducted in the 1960s in Alameda County, California, identified a handful of habits that promoted longevity. One of those habits was getting seven to eight hours of sleep per night.

After a good night's sleep, you awake feeling rested and ready to take on the challenges of the day. You know the feeling—but it happens all too rarely, it seems. This rested feeling is a product of the amount of time you've been sleeping, the quality of your sleep, and the amount of time you spend in each of the sleep stages.

Your body may be resting, but your brain is busy, while you're snoozing. During deep sleep, your brain is generating creative ideas, storing memories, and enhancing your ability to learn new tasks. Your brain is also producing growth hormones, sex hormones, and hunger-controlling hormones. It's also generating infection-fighting proteins and enhancing your mood, reducing your risk for depression. It's a full slate of jobs and it takes time to get them done.

How much sleep do you need? Your needs change over the course of your lifetime. Young children not only need more sleep than adults, they also spend more of their sleep time in deep sleep. By adolescence, the amount of time spent in the deep stages of sleep starts to drop, and by middle age we may be spending less than 5 percent of our sleep in deep-stage sleep. In addition to this natural process of decreasing deep-sleep time, medical problems and certain medications can disrupt sleep.

The Stages of Sleep

Sleep is divided into two main stages: REM sleep (Rapid Eye Movement) and non-REM sleep. Non-REM sleep gets further broken down into four stages, ranging from light to ever-deepening sleep. The last two stages of non-REM sleep, stages three and four, are especially important. They're considered the deep stages of sleep, and it's difficult to arouse a sleeper in these stages.

When doctors talk about *restorative* sleep, they're referring to the amount of time spent in stages 3 and 4. Here's where that restful, refreshed feeling originates. You can sleep intermittently for hours, but not until you have a few cycles of stage three and four sleep do you wake up feeling refreshed. This is why medical residents and parents of newborns are perpetually fatigued, as well as men with prostate problems who have to get up multiple times a night to urinate.

The restorative sleep stages naturally diminish with age, but in this chapter we'll discuss what you can do to optimize your restful sleep—and enhance your health span in the process.

Falling Asleep

Try as hard as you might, you can only hold off sleep for so long. That's because your brain produces a number of chemicals, including adenosine and melatonin, that induce sleep, much like the poppy fields that put Dorothy and her companions to sleep in the *Wizard of Oz*.

Melatonin is a hormone made by a part of the brain called the pineal gland. Scientists think that melatonin may help our sleep cycle by letting our bodies know when it's time to go to sleep and when it's time to wake up. Melatonin release generally starts when the sun goes down; it's also produced in early afternoon, and that's when many of us experience that post-lunch stupor. Melatonin supplements are sometimes used by people with insomnia to help them sleep and may be particularly useful as we age—more about this later in the chapter!

Sleep Deprivation: Risky Business

Chronic sleep deprivation decreases your life span. It has serious, negative consequences for your health and increases your risk of specific medical conditions. Researchers continue to study just how sleep is implicated in various diseases. They do know, however, that sleep disorders play a role in developing ...

- ◆ Cardiovascular disease.
- ◆ Increased blood inflammation.
- ◆ Diabetes and pre-diabetes.
- ◆ Obesity and food cravings.
- ◆ Depression and other mood changes.

◆ Fibromyalgia and other aches and pains.

◆ Higher rate of infections and reduced response to some vaccinations.

◆ Hormone imbalances.

Doctors' Orders _____

Don't get behind the wheel, if you're tired—it is the same as driving when you are drunk! According to the National Transportation Safety Board, tired drivers cause 100,000 accidents per year, leading to 1,500 deaths. Sleep-deprived drivers are at high risk of having an accident. One study found that these drivers drove as if they had an alcohol level of 0.05 percent. Warning signs of driver fatigue include daydreaming while on the road, driving over the center line, excessive yawning, feeling impatient, feeling stiff, heavy eyes, and reacting slowly.

Sleep Disorders

Do you have a sleep disorder? Taking more than 30 minutes to fall asleep at night, or waking frequently during the night, may be signs of *insomnia*. There is more to insomnia than just nighttime problems, however. You might feel excessively sleepy or tired during the day, have headaches, be irritable, have difficulty concentrating, or become forgetful. When you can't sleep, you start to worry about not sleeping—you become anxious.

There's a real concern here, and that's the increased chance of accidents at work or while driving. Insomnia can affect your decision-making abilities, and this could mean trouble. If any of these symptoms describe you, talk to your doctor about them. There is help available for sleep disorders.

def•i•ni•tion _____

Insomnia is defined by the International Classification of Sleep Disorders as difficulty falling asleep or staying asleep, or the inability to achieve restful sleep, despite adequate time in bed, in addition to daytime complaints.

For many people, insomnia begins during a period of stress or imbalance in their lives. If insomnia is temporary, it's called *acute insomnia*. If not attended to, insomnia can then develop into a chronic pattern, which means you have difficulty sleeping more than three nights a week over a time frame of more than a month. About one third of adults will have insomnia at some point, and about 10 to 15 percent of adults have chronic or severe insomnia. Chronic insomnia affects more women than men and becomes more common as you age.

Sleep Stealers

While sleep deprivation can increase your risk of developing certain medical conditions, the opposite is also true. There's a multitude of conditions that can carry insomnia along with them.

In some cases, pain is the factor that disrupts your sleep. This is the case with arthritis and other musculoskeletal diseases, such as fibromyalgia. Sometimes, however, the pain is the result of the condition that's keeping you from a restful night. If you awaken in the morning with a sore jaw, the pain you feel may be the result of a condition known as bruxism—teeth grinding. As you grind away during the night, you are also losing quality sleep time. A special nightguard, worn in your mouth as you sleep, can control bruxism. Check with your dentist if you think you might be grinding your teeth.

Cardiovascular disease, including heart disease, angina, and congestive heart failure, is a major sleep stealer. Lung disorders, such as asthma and emphysema, can interfere with your sleep. Struggling for breath and nighttime coughing make sleep difficult, if not nearly impossible.

Words to the Wise

Snoring got you down? Solutions may include treatment of sinus problems, treatment of any diagnosed sleep apnea, and weight loss. If none of those are helpful, ear plugs and/or separate sleeping areas may be a solution. In fact, according to some in the real estate business, separate sleeping areas, also known as snoring rooms, are now one of the hottest selling points in new luxury homes.

The discomfort of intestinal disorders, including irritable bowel syndrome and heartburn, can keep you tossing and turning and eventually can drive you out of the bedroom and into the bathroom, seeking relief from the symptoms. Urinary tract disorders provide another source of trips to the bathroom at night.

For men, prostate gland enlargement is a primary cause of nighttime bathroom treks. For many women, menopause brings hot flashes, night sweats, and insomnia.

Thyroid disorders, especially hyperthyroidism, will interfere with your sleep, as will neurological disorders, including Parkinson's and Alzheimer's. Mental health conditions that cause insomnia include depression, anxiety, stress, and schizophrenia.

The good news here is that in treating the specific medical condition, you will be treating the cause of your insomnia. You don't have to accept sleeplessness as a permanent state.

Other Spoilers

In addition to medical conditions, other things can keep you from a good night's sleep:

♦ *Prescription medications:* Many prescription medications can cause or worsen insomnia. These meds include decongestants, stimulants (such as Ritalin), some antidepressants, thyroid medications, bronchodilators (asthma medications), beta blockers, and steroids. Always read the labels carefully to see what common side effects there may be from your meds. If you have questions, your pharmacist is trained to answer those questions.

♦ *Alcohol:* Although alcohol seems to produce a drowsy state, it actually reduces deep-stage and REM sleep and increases the likelihood of nocturnal awakenings. If you're having difficulty sleeping, alcohol can compound the problem. So nix on the nightcap!

♦ *Caffeine:* Caffeine can interfere with your ability to fall asleep for up to eight hours. This happens because caffeine can block the chemical adenosine from producing its sleep-inducing effects. If you enjoy a cup of coffee or tea after dinner, consider switching to decaf.

♦ *Nicotine:* If you needed one more reason to quit smoking, this is it. Nicotine can reduce your deep-stage sleep, and nicotine withdrawal in the wee hours of the morning can cause you to wake up, craving a cigarette, unable to return to sleep.

♦ *Excessive stimulation:* Even a healthful practice, such as exercising, should be done earlier in the day. It takes time for your body to wind down after a strenuous workout. To encourage sleep, you need to focus on relaxing activities, not on pumping iron. Also, exercise may reduce the melatonin secretion that helps in falling asleep.

Diagnosing Sleep Disorders

Okay, you think you're pretty healthy, but you still can't sleep. What to do? Get out a sheet of paper and prepare to take notes! You're going to pinpoint where your sleep problem lies. For the next week or two, you're going to keep a sleep diary.

Keeping a Sleep Diary

When trying to sort out what's causing your insomnia, keeping a sleep diary for one or two weeks can help show you where your sleep problem lies. For your sleep diary, you'll consider sleep and factors that impact your sleep. You're going to be focusing on the numbers, so each day should follow the same format. For the first section, write down the time you went to bed, how long it took to fall asleep (you'll need to estimate this, of course), and the time you woke up in the morning. If you woke up during the night, how many times? Also, try to figure out what caused you to wake up. Write down how long it took you to go back to sleep. (Again, you'll have to estimate.)

The next section has to do with other factors. If you had any physical symptoms or sensations while in bed, describe them. For example, were your legs restless? Did you have heartburn?

If you're a napper, jot down the number and length of naps you took during the day. Also, if you consumed alcohol, caffeine, nicotine, or recreational drugs, write down how much and when. This is not the time to hold back. Be truthful.

Write down the times you exercised, along with the length, amount, and type.

Finally, list the prescription or over-the-counter meds you take and the times you take them. After a week or two, you'll have a good snapshot of your sleep patterns.

Here's a sample sleep diary format you can use:

The time you go to sleep _____

The amount of time it takes to fall asleep _____

The time you wake up _____

The number of times you woke up while sleeping _____;
length of time you were awake _____; what it was that woke you up

_____

Physical symptoms or sensations you have while in bed _____

_____

The number and amount of naps you took _____

Consumption of the following; include amount and time at which it was consumed:

   Alcohol _____

Caffeine _____

Nicotine _____

Recreational drugs _____

The amount and type of exercise you did _____;

time of exercise _____

Prescription meds you took and when you took them _____

_____

Over-the-counter meds you took and when you took them _____

_____

Sleep Evaluation

If you have chronic insomnia that is happening more than a couple of times a week and is negatively impacting your health, your doctor will probably pursue workup and treatment. One of the first steps is to keep a sleep diary, as we've just described; once you've completed that, it's time to meet with your doctor, who may order a sleep study for you. This is usually done overnight in a sleep lab. The goal here is to first rule out any undiagnosed medical problems that might be causing your insomnia. Once these are treated, sleep often improves and no further treatment for insomnia is needed. If your insomnia is the result of some disruptive sleep habits you've developed, you'll receive some instruction in how to overcome them and get back on track to a restful night's sleep.

> **Words to the Wise**
>
> Benjamin Franklin said that "Fatigue is the best pillow." Exercising regularly, having a daily routine, and avoiding excessive napping helps create a sound sleep.

Mind over Pillow

Once insomnia sets in, many people develop anxiety about their ability to sleep normally again. This anxiety can set off a vicious cycle of disrupted sleep and fearful thinking and worrying. Cognitive/behavioral therapy (CBT) is extremely helpful here. In CBT, you learn how to use your mind to effect changes in your behavior and get back to the business of sound sleeping. Your physician can recommend or refer you to a licensed psychotherapist who will guide you through the CBT process.

Anxiety is the enemy of sleep. CBT teaches you how to relax your body to control that anxiety. CBT can help you reframe your thinking. It can replace distorted thinking and fear about sleep with more empowering self-talk. This positive self-talk helps you create what *you* want, instead of feeling victimized by the worries of your fretful mind.

Meditation, guided imagery, progressive muscle relaxation, deep-breathing exercises, and bio-feedback are other forms of relaxation therapy. When your body and mind are at ease, worry has no place to enter. Being present in the moment and focusing on your body will help you achieve that relaxation that leads to good sleep.

> ### Words to the Wise
>
> Sound and healthy sleep is a habit that can be learned with a little practice. Try to get at least 30 minutes of exposure to natural sunlight during the day. Avoid daytime napping. Avoid caffeine, alcohol, nicotine, and exercise in the later parts of the evening. Develop a restful ritual before your bedtime (soothing music, warm bath, chamomile tea, etc.) Setting a regular sleep schedule is important, and so is keeping your bedroom quiet, cool, and restful. If you find that you can't fall asleep after 15 minutes in bed, get up and go do something boring. Return to bed when you feel sleepy again.

Prescription Meds

If your insomnia hasn't responded to your best efforts, you and your doctor may decide to consider prescription medications to help you sleep. When used judiciously, they can be a godsend. Ideally, these medications should be for *short-term use only*. Many people, however, have chronic insomnia and may need meds for long periods of time. Fortunately, many of these drugs, such as Ambien CR, Lunesta, and Rozerem, are now approved by the FDA for long-term use. Use them wisely: try to limit their use to several times per week or less, never exceed recommended doses, and avoid taking them with other mood-altering medications and substances, including anxiety meds, pain pills, or alcohol.

Benzodiazepine Sleeping Meds

These meds include Restoril, Halcion, Ativan, Dalmane, and others. They work by mimicking a chemical in your central nervous system. This chemical, gamma-aminobutyric acid (GABA), helps calm you, relax you, and put you to sleep. These drugs came on the market in the 1960s and became popular for sleep in the 1980s, replacing barbiturates as sleeping pills. They're less popular now because of many other alternatives. These drugs can cause dependence pretty quickly. Please note that these drugs have been associated with a higher incidence of falls and hip fractures the day after they are taken; they should be used with caution in the elderly.

Non-Benzodiazepine Sleeping Meds

These new drugs have been available since early 2000 and are also felt to work by binding to GABA receptors. All of these medications have their good points, as well as their shortcomings. Some will help you fall asleep quickly. They are useful if being unable to fall asleep is your main problem. They aren't useful for keeping you asleep for your full eight hours, however. These drugs are FDA–approved for short-term use only. Ambien and Sonata fall into this category. Sonata is even shorter-acting than Ambien but doesn't generally leave you feeling groggy the next morning.

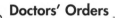

Doctors' Orders

Sedating antidepressants, such as Elavil and Trazodone, are sometimes used to help people sleep. Unfortunately, there is little evidence for their effectiveness for treating insomnia.

Lunesta is a longer-acting drug and should only be used if you are able to spend a full eight hours in bed. Another drug with longer-acting capabilities is Ambien CR, a newer and longer-acting version of Ambien. Rozerem is a melatonin-like drug that may be useful for people who have difficulty falling asleep, but it may not help you to stay asleep. Unlike the others, abuse potential with Rozerem is felt to be minimal.

Over-the-Counter Products

Sedating antihistamines are often used by folks with insomnia. Benadryl and doxylamine are approved by the FDA for sleep, but they have side effects, including dizziness, fatigue, and morning hangover. They have not been well studied for insomnia, their safety profile is unclear, and they often stop working for people who take them chronically.

Alternative Therapies and Supplements

If you prefer to choose natural products to induce sleep, you have some options that include hormones, herbs, and fragrance. Keep in mind that herbs can interact with many medicines, both prescription and over-the-counter, and they also come with their own set of side effects. Check with your doctor before starting any herbal products.

Melatonin decreases the amount of time it takes to fall asleep and may improve the overall quality of sleep. The recommended dose is 1 to 3 mg; most sleep doctors recommend taking it two to three hours before bedtime. It also helps your immune system and can ward off headaches. Some people also use melatonin to prevent jet lag.

Valerian is an herb that has been widely used for insomnia, especially for people with chronic insomnia. It may work by interacting with GABA receptors, in much the same way prescription meds do. It may take several weeks to take full effect, so it is not suitable for treatment of acute insomnia. The most typical dose used is 600 mg per day.

Kava-Kava is an herbal remedy made from the roots of the plant *Piper methysticum*. It has been used for ceremonial purposes for thousands of years in Polynesia, and because of its antianxiety properties, has been sold as an anxiety and sleep aid in the West. However, because of reports of severe liver toxicity, it has recently been banned in several European countries. The FDA has also issued a consumer advisory here in the United States but has not yet banned its sale.

Aromatherapy is the ancient practice of using essential oils from plants and flowers to evoke relaxation, mental clarity, and peace. Scents and smells can evoke powerful feelings and physical responses for many of us. The scent of lavender oil has often been used for calming, and the aroma of apples may reduce the stress response. At the very least, aromatherapy is pleasant to the senses and creates a warm and inviting atmosphere.

The Least You Need to Know

- Insomnia can lead to medical conditions that can shorten the life span.
- Many internal and external factors can lead to sleep disorders.
- Consult with your doctor if you are having significant problems sleeping to determine the cause of your insomnia.
- Work with your physician on a treatment plan for your insomnia.
- Create regular sleep habits and a good sleep environment.
- Use sleeping pills only when all else fails.

Chapter 9

Touch, Connection, and Sex

In This Chapter

- ◆ Life-giving touch
- ◆ Making social connections
- ◆ The health benefits of having a pet
- ◆ Nature's healing powers
- ◆ Maintaining sexual health
- ◆ Keeping the fires burning at any age

We are social creatures, meant to interact and live with others of our species. Increasing and strengthening social connections with family, neighbors, friends, and even nature itself can help us live longer, healthier lives. In this chapter, you'll explore ways to enhance your connection with your surroundings and learn life-changing techniques to enhance your longevity and health span.

The Power of Human Touch and Connection

In our eternal quest for the fountain of youth, we exercise, eat well, take our medications, and see our doctors regularly. But what if a part of your prescription to good health and long life was to connect deeply to what surrounds you?

Touch and Thriving

We human beings have five senses, but only one has been found to be essential to human survival. The sense of touch, the feel of skin upon skin, is that sense. Touch is vitally important to our well-being.

Orphanages in World War II (and more recent wars as well) are a testimony to the power of touch on human survival. These babies, left alone in their cribs for extended periods of time, had an increased rate of mortality, attributed to lack of human touch. Today we know that infants in preemie wards fare better when held by a human being for a few hours each day.

Longevity Facts _____

In the famous experiments by scientist Harry Harlow in the 1950s on the importance of touch, newborn monkeys were given a choice of a soft terrycloth or a wire "surrogate mother." The monkeys consistently chose the terrycloth mother—even when given an option between the soft mother and food. The newborn monkeys needed the feel of a mother more than they needed food. The need for touch is universal and crosses all borders and boundaries.

Touch has been linked to many health benefits—from enhanced growth for preterm infants, to decreased pain, increased immunity, enhanced alertness, and improved performance for the rest of us. It is felt that many of these health benefits arise from reduced levels of stress hormones in the body, in those receiving the touch.

Interestingly enough, in international studies done evaluating the frequency of touch, the United States and Great Britain were the two countries with the least amount of human touch occurring in social interactions. The sick and the elderly in our society are at greatest risk for decreased touch, in part because of their greater risk of social isolation.

Massage Therapy

Massage therapy is a technique that incorporates the power of human touch into the healing process. Massage has been used as a healing therapy for thousands of years. We know it was used in the ancient cultures of India, Egypt, China, and Rome. Today, there are at least 80 different types of massage techniques performed in the

United States. These include Swedish massage, deep tissue massage, shiatsu massage, and trigger point massage. These various massages differ in the types and locations of pressures applied to the body.

def•i•ni•tion

> **Massage therapy** is a term used to define a process in which therapists press, rub, and manipulate muscles and soft tissues with pressure from their hands or other parts of their body. Massage is used to decrease pain and relax the soft tissues and muscles, with the typical massage session lasting anywhere from 30 minutes to 1 hour.

Scientists feel that massage therapy may work by enhancing relaxation and decreasing stress. Massaging may provide stimulation that blocks the pain signals that are sent to the brain. It may also trigger the release of chemicals that help in decreasing pain—serotonin and endorphins. Massage also may cause mechanical changes in the body that reduce inflammation and stimulate the flow of lymph fluid throughout the body.

About 5 percent of the American population uses massage therapy. It is most commonly used for painful musculoskeletal conditions, sports injuries, to reduce stress, increase relaxation, and for general wellness. In the hands of a good practitioner, it is a relatively safe healing technique—choose a licensed massage therapist (LMT) or a certified massage therapist (CMT).

However, the following people may have complications from massage therapy and should talk to their physician prior to getting a massage:

◆ Those on blood thinners, such as Coumadin. Massage may cause excessive bruising or bleeding in these cases.

◆ People with a blood clot, such as a deep vein thrombosis (DVT). Massage may cause the clot to break off and travel to the lungs.

◆ Those with weak bones, severe osteoporosis, or a fracture. Massage may lead to broken bones.

◆ People with an open or healing wound or other skin breakdown. Massage may lead to increased skin breakdown and infection.

Human Connection: Volunteering for Vitality

Volunteering is one of the most beneficial activities you can take up at various stages in your life. The altruistic aspect is a great reason to volunteer your time or services to a cause that inspires you. Volunteering helps your community, provides resources that could not otherwise be accessed, and can help solve social problems.

In addition, volunteering has been shown in many studies to be of great benefit to the health of those who volunteer their time or energy. Research has shown that volunteering …

◆ Enhances the social networks of the volunteers. People with strong social networks have been shown to have reduced risks of depression, less heart disease, and fewer health risk factors.

◆ Can improve self-esteem and increase endorphin production in the brain (the "happy chemical").

◆ Reduces mortality. A University of Michigan study showed that people who volunteered in one organization for 40 hours or less in one year lived longer than those who did not volunteer. The protective effects of volunteering are greatest for those who have low levels of social interaction.

◆ Leads to better health and sense of well-being in the person who volunteers.

> **Longevity Facts**
>
> A 10-year study of the physical health and social activities of 2,700 men in Tecumseh, Michigan, found that those who did regular volunteer work had death rates two and a half times lower than those who didn't.

◆ Gives people social interaction and social identities. This creates the opportunity to develop new close interpersonal relationships and leads to a strengthened sense of identity.

There are so many benefits associated with volunteering. It's difficult to come up with any other activity that positively impacts so many people on so many levels.

Anecdotal evidence of the benefits of volunteering abound. Consider Samantha, a 71-year-old female with few friends and whose only daughter lived in another state. She was blessed by a long marriage and financial security but was unable to combat long-standing depression despite therapy and medications. She was advised by her physician to start volunteering. When she returned to her doctor six months later, she had a renewed sense of vitality and purpose: "Doctor, the volunteering helped me shift my focus from myself and what I don't have to what I can do for others to help in their problems. This has shifted my entire frame of thinking. I am happy for the first time in years!"

You can look to your own community for opportunities to engage your body and your mind in this rewarding activity. Pick up the phone and align yourself with your favorite cause, be it volunteering in the local hospital, food bank, women's shelter, animal shelter, or church. Your body will thank you. Happiness is a prime asset for your health span, as well as your life span.

Expanding Connections: Pets and Companion Animals

Yes, your dog Fido is the joy of your life, and you could not imagine your home without the delightful presence of your cat Muffy. But did you know that not only are they providing you much-needed companionship, laughter, love, and attention, but they are also keeping you healthy? Pets are great for the mind, reduce depression, help the cardiovascular system, and provide great company in their spare time.

Many studies have been done on the relationship of companion animals and the health of their human owners. Some fascinating study outcomes include the following:

◆ Pets can decrease your blood pressure. One study showed significant decreases in blood pressure when people petted their animals, as opposed to reading aloud. Other studies showed that just the presence of a pet in the room can decrease heart rate and blood pressure.

◆ Pets may calm you down more than your spouse does! Studies showed that when people were stressed by the presence of their spouse in the room, the presence of their pet helped calm their blood pressure and heart rate and improved their ability to perform tasks.

◆ Pet owners survive a heart attack better than those who do not have pets. One-year survival rates after a heart attack were higher in pet owners than those who did not have a pet.

◆ Pets can reduce depression. Pet visits have been shown to reduce anxiety about hospital stays and reduce depression in nursing homes.

So if you are in a stage of your life where you are living independently, are able to take care of another living being, and are alone, why not consider a pet? The health benefits may be immeasurable—the new pet may become your personal secret to longevity!

Creating Family: They're All Around You

With the many studies that have been conducted on social ties and isolation, we now know that social isolation leads to illness. We further know that having close friends decreases the incidence of depression, reduces death from heart disease, and improves overall health. It makes sense for those who want to live a long and fulfilling life to create a strong social network. These social ties will be the support structure that will help through tough times and illness. These friends will be able to support you in your life, and giving them support will give additional meaning to your life.

Where do you find your friends? They exist all around you. You may go to the nearest animal shelter and pick out a furry friend. You may decide to volunteer at the local hospital for two hours a week. You could serve food at the local food bank. You could knit blankets for the local hospital or charity. You could be a mentor for an under-privileged youth. You could join a cooking or exercise class at your local community center. All of these activities provide ample opportunities for friendships and mean-ingful interaction.

There is a saying, "Friends are family you choose." Choose to have a rich, fulfilling life, and you will discover that friends are all around you.

Nature Connections

How about a prescription for a weekend trip to the campgrounds for your fatigue? Or a prescription for gardening to reduce your stress? Believe it or not, these are not far-fetched health remedies and at times may work better than prescription pills. Until the urbanization of the last 200 years, humans had a close relationship with nature. Not surprisingly, science is finding that nature is closely tied to our healing process. We derive numerous health benefits from living in harmony and contact with nature.

> **Words to the Wise**
>
> For optimum health, do what our ancestors knew instinctively: love the earth, and it will help sustain and support your health.

Research has shown that viewing nature speeds recovery from illness. Being outside has been shown to reduce mental fatigue, decrease irritabil-ity, increase problem-solving abilities, and improve concentration. Anyone who has gone camping over the weekend or for a simple walk through the woods can attest to this. For those who can't get away to experience nature, gardening has been shown to decrease stress and improve nurturing characteristics. And if you can't or don't like to garden, get a house plant. Caring for another life, even if it's a green one, has been shown to improve mood and well-being—and a plant can also improve your air quality, to boot!

Sex and Your Health

Here is the longevity secret you have been waiting to have your doctors tell you: *sex is great for your health!* Not only does it help keep you healthy, but there is evidence that frequent sex increases longevity. Of course, it is one of the most fun human activities, and most of us don't need a medical excuse to have sex. But for those of you who need some arm-twisting to encourage you, here are some important reasons why you should have sex:

◆ Sex may reduce pain. During orgasm, the brain releases the chemical oxytocin, which then may help release endorphins into the body. These endorphins may help reduce migraines, pain, arthritis, and menstrual cramps in women.

◆ It may decrease the incidence of prostate cancer. The *British Journal of Urology* online reported in 2003 on a study that found that men in their 20s could reduce their chances of prostate cancer by a third by ejaculating more than five times a week.

◆ Sex may prevent illnesses such as the cold and flu. A Wilkes University study, made available in 1999, found that people who have sex one or two times a week had higher levels of Immunoglobulin A, a chemical that boosts immunity in the body.

> **Doctors' Orders**
>
> Unprotected sex is only safe in a monogamous relationship where both partners have tested negative for STDs.

◆ It prolongs life. A study reported in the 1997 *British Medical Journal* followed 1,000 men over 10 years and found that men who had a higher frequency of orgasm had half the death rate compared with those who had fewer orgasms.

◆ Sex burns calories. An energetic sexual encounter can burn off around 200 calories.

◆ It gives your muscles a workout. Muscles in the pubococcygeal area (the ones that help bladder control) are strengthened during sex. Muscles in the back, thighs, gluteus, abdomen, and arms can also get a good workout during sex.

That's great, you say, and you do remember the days of uninhibited sex, passionate sex, wild sex, and endless sex. But you're older now, and the sex drive declines with age. Here's where it's helpful to remember that sex in maturity is a self-fulfilling prophecy to a certain extent. Taking care of your body, living your life as a confident sexual being, and continuing to adapt to your body's needs are the keys to having a powerful sex life at all ages.

Sexual intimacy is one of life's most precious gifts. Love and sex don't have to fall by the wayside as you grow older. In fact, with all that fuss and worry gone, sex can be downright liberating. Enjoy sex—and live healthier and longer!

Sexual Dysfunction in Men

Although men may not talk about it much with their buddies, much less their sexual partners, sexual dysfunction is common in men over the age of 40. The most common sexual problem in males is erectile dysfunction (ED), defined as inability to have an erection sufficient for orgasm or penetration. Other common problems include intimacy problems (problems in the sexual relationship arising from relationship issues) and premature ejaculation.

Longevity Facts _____

A Harvard health study looked at 30,000 men to determine various factors that contributed to ED. Researchers found that the lifestyles that most helped maintain erectile functioning were physical activity and leanness, and those that were physically active had a 30 percent lower risk of ED than those who weren't. Smoking, alcohol consumption, and television viewing were the activities most strongly associated with increased ED. Other research shows that exercise leads to increased flexibility and coordination and a better sense of self-esteem.

The phosphodiesterase inhibitors—medications in the Viagra category—have revolutionized the treatment of ED. These are medications that help improve the blood supply to the penis and help strengthen the erection. They need to be taken 30 minutes to 1 hour before intercourse. If you take nitrate medications for heart disease, however, then you should not use these medications.

A certain proportion of men will have low levels of testosterone, and if this is the case, testosterone supplementation may help erectile functioning.

Besides Viagra, treatment for erectile dysfunction includes urological aids such as penile pumps, implants, suppositories, and injections. A penile pump is a cylindrical device with a manual or motorized pump to create suction. It is placed over the penis. As the apparatus creates a vacuum around the penis, blood is drawn into the penis, helping it to become engorged. This mechanical suction helps to achieve an erection.

Penile implants are surgically placed inside the penis for men suffering from complete impotence. An implanted pump in the groin or scrotum is manipulated by hand—this pump is attached to a reservoir and fills cylinders placed in the penis to achieve an erection. The erection can be controlled in terms of duration, amount, and timing.

When used, penile suppositories and injections stimulate an immediate erection.

Sexual Dysfunction in Women

Sexual dysfunction in women can be due to many issues, and the source of a low libido (low sex drive) can be hard to pinpoint. Low libido in women may be caused by heart disease, depression, thyroid conditions, diabetes, or atrophic vaginitis. Get a checkup if you have a low libido to rule out physical causes. Some other common issues that cause a low libido include:

◆ Some women are very estrogen-driven, or more likely, testosterone-driven. As they get older and the levels of these hormones decline, so can their libido. Low levels of estrogen lead to atrophic vaginitis, or a dry vagina. This can make sex less pleasurable and occasionally painful. Vaginal lubrication can also decrease with aging and hormonal changes. If sex stops feeling good, women are not as likely to seek it out.

◆ Relationship and intimacy issues play a big role in determining libido. If a woman is not happy with her sexual partner, her libido will go down the drain.

◆ Psychological stress will undermine a healthy libido. Depression needs to be treated if it is present.

Just as with men, there is help available for treating sexual dysfunction in women. Estrogen replacement therapy can be beneficial in decreasing hot flashes, mood swings, and reversing atrophic vaginitis (dry, thinning vagina) after menopause. It comes in the form of pills, rings, patches, and topical creams.

For a failing libido in women, however, testosterone replacement appears to work even better than estrogen. Women have small levels of testosterone produced naturally in their bodies, and these levels decline with age, decreasing the libido. A small dose of testosterone can be beneficial in perking up the libido in some women. Over-supplementation of testosterone in women can have side effects, including facial hair, deepening of the voice, and enlargement of the clitoris. There are no long-term studies looking at the safety of testosterone supplementation in women, so if you give testosterone a try, use it at the lowest possible dose and for the shortest period of time needed.

> **Doctors' Orders** _____
>
> If your libido does not get a boost with hormones, get checked out for stress or depression and get treated for it, if necessary.

Some women prefer bioidentical hormones—hormones that are closer to what the body naturally produces. Just because a hormone is bioidentical, however, does not mean that it is better for you or comes with fewer risks. It is the hormone itself that causes the side effects of increased cancer and heart disease—not the fact that it is artificial or natural. There are no studies that show that bioidentical hormones are safer, so take them at your own risk.

Some women may find that it's harder to achieve an orgasm as they get older. If this describes you, then you may benefit from using a vibrator as part of your foreplay; this can help you to increase lubrication and achieve a more powerful orgasm. Similarly, a medical device called a clitoral suction device can be beneficial in pulling the blood supply to the surface of the clitoris and enhancing sensation and orgasm during sex.

Enhancing Sexual Intimacy

So how do you have a phenomenal sex life at any age? Take the following steps to ensure great sexual functioning:

◆ Control diseases such as diabetes, high cholesterol, hypertension, and obesity—these lead to sexual dysfunction.

◆ Address physical problems such as back pain, atrophic vaginitis, or ED with your doctor. Most men over 50 will have some degree of ED. Get treated for this.

◆ Eat a healthy diet and get eight hours of sleep a night.

◆ Get plenty of exercise. Aerobic exercise has been shown to enhance blood supply to the genitalia, enhancing the orgasmic response.

◆ Reinvent yourself as a sexual being. Focus on self-love and self-esteem. Sex is not only for perfectly proportioned 20-year-olds.

◆ Bring sexual intimacy back into your relationship—if you don't use it, you lose it! Continue to focus on communicating effectively with your partner. Your words are your ultimate sex tool!

◆ Learn something new. Make allowances for your aging body—discover new positions and experiment with sexual aids. Women will need more time with foreplay. And lubrication is the key to smooth sex!

There are many secrets to enhancing intimacy, but here are five that will help you along your way:

1. Deep breathing in the spoon position. Lie down back to stomach, hold your partner, and breathe together for five minutes. This brings amazing intimacy into the partnership, without any stress of the eventual outcome.

2. Focus on the pleasure, not on the goal—it really doesn't matter if one of you does not reach orgasm all the time. The pleasure that you derive from sexual intimacy should be the goal. Mutual orgasms are just icing on the cake.

3. Lock your eyes during intimacy. Look deeply into each other's eyes when you are in a face-to-face position, and do not look away. Continue to do this until orgasm.

4. Use sex toys. The hands get more arthritic, the penis gets softer, and the female orgasm takes longer. Start using vibrators as a part of your normal foreplay.

5. Learn the male and female kegels and use them during intercourse. Isolate the muscles that stop urination by trying to stop your urinary flow. When you know which muscles to isolate, do three sets of 10 clenches daily. For women, this enhances vaginal muscle tone and the quality of the female orgasm and reduces urinary incontinence. For men, it is useful to prevent premature ejaculation—just clench and unclench the same muscles during intercourse when getting too close to orgasm.

Longevity Facts

Good sex contributes to long life. To enhance your longevity, recreate the romance in your life and reap the benefits of a healthy, sexual relationship!

Deep intimacy won't happen without love. This means love of yourself, love of your body, love of your partner, and love of the moment. Be present, be loving, and don't forget to laugh!

The Least You Need to Know

◆ Social connections lead to decreased illness and enhance longevity.

◆ Human touch is essential for survival.

◆ Volunteering has numerous health benefits.

◆ Pets are great companions—and help you stay healthy!

◆ You can learn to make a network of friends no matter what stage of life you're in.

◆ Frequent sex helps you live better, longer! There is much you can do to enhance your sexual intimacy as you age.

Part 3

Longevity and Health: Knowledge Is Power

Now we take a look at what you can do to prevent or minimize the diseases that commonly cause disability and shorten life span for many Americans. Although chronic disease such as heart disease, diabetes, and arthritis are common as we age, it's a myth to think that we don't have a say in preventing or delaying their onset. In fact, there's *a lot* you can do to prevent disease and disability and maintain vibrant good health as you age—this is referred to as *successful aging*. In this part, you find a road map for navigating this territory. You also get the latest information on hormone and dermatologic treatments for the aging boomer.

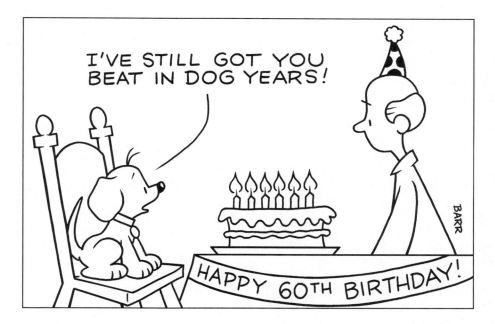

Chapter 10

Your Healthy Heart

In This Chapter

◆ Lowering your risk for heart disease

◆ Good numbers = long life

◆ Eating your way to heart health

◆ Heart disease in men versus women

◆ Knowledge is power: heart screenings

◆ Medications that help your heart

The human heart—designed to last over 75 years. Optimally? Over 100! Yet according to the Centers for Disease Control (CDC), heart disease is the leading cause of death for both men and women, claiming around 700,000 victims in this country each year. If you want to live long, preventing heart disease is vitally important to your goal. In this chapter, you'll learn how to assess your risk, along with preventive measures you can take to enjoy a healthy life span.

Prevention Is Primary

Studies have shown that, even if you don't have pre-existing heart disease, lowering high blood pressure and cholesterol can reduce your risk of developing this condition. Also, for those who do have existing heart disease, lowering high cholesterol and high blood pressure can reduce the risk of dying from heart disease, having a nonfatal heart attack, or needing heart surgery or angioplasty. About 30 percent of adults aged 20 and older have high blood pressure, and 17 percent of adults aged 20 and older have high cholesterol.

Heart Attack

Sudden cardiac death is often the first sign of heart disease. Approximately 400,000 deaths each year are the result of sudden heart attacks. Thus, symptoms of heart disease may be subtle, and the first major event may lead to death. The longevity take-home here is to know and reduce your cardiovascular risk factors early, and to acquaint yourself with the signs and symptoms of heart disease.

The classic symptoms of a heart attack may feel like crushing chest pain that occurs at the center of the chest and radiates to the jaw or left arm. Some patients also describe this as "an elephant sitting on my chest." These are the typical signs, but there are also some subtle signs and symptoms of a heart attack that can include the following:

◆ Difficulty breathing

◆ Lightheadedness

◆ Palpitations or heart fluttering

◆ An irregular heartbeat

◆ Feeling faint

◆ Indigestion

◆ Sense of impending doom

◆ Unusual fatigue with exercise

◆ Pain in upper back, jaw, or neck

◆ Sweating

◆ Nausea

Women in particular are much more likely to have atypical symptoms of heart disease. If you experience any of these symptoms and they are not going away, call 911. If you have questions, discuss them with your doctor.

Risk Factors: Know Your Numbers

There are many risk factors for heart or *coronary artery disease*, but the top six are smoking, high blood pressure, high cholesterol, diabetes, obesity, and physical inactivity. According to the CDC, in 2003, 37 percent of adults reported having two or more of these six risk factors for heart disease or stroke. If you have two or more risk factors, then addressing and correcting them may very well add many years to your life.

def•i•ni•tion

> **Coronary artery disease,** also known as atherosclerosis, refers to blockage in the arteries that supply blood to the heart muscle. These blockages, also called plaque, are caused by smoking, diabetes, high blood pressure, high cholesterol, and inactivity. They can decrease or prevent blood flow to the region of the heart supplied by the artery. Coronary artery disease is the leading cause of death for both men and women in the United States.

Peripheral artery disease (PAD) is a condition similar to coronary artery disease. In PAD, fatty deposits build up in the inner linings of the artery walls, restricting blood circulation. This can occur in arteries leading to the kidneys, stomach, arms, legs, and feet. Peripheral arterial disease affects 8 million adults in the United States. Longevity secret? Don't smoke—this raises your risk of PAD three-and-a-half-fold.

You want to do all you can to decrease your risk of heart disease, but you are not sure if you fall into the high risk categories. How do you find out? Know your numbers—the American Heart Association (AHA) recommends keeping track of your blood pressure, blood lipids, and blood sugar.

Smoking

People who smoke have a two to four times greater risk of developing heart and vascular disease compared to those who don't smoke. Cigars, pipes, and secondhand smoke also increase the risk of developing heart disease—though not as much as smoking cigarettes.

Cigarette smoking accelerates the accumulation of plaque in arteries—it accelerates atherosclerosis. It also increases the levels of blood-clotting factors, such as fibrinogen. Nicotine raises blood pressure and the carbon monoxide produced by smoking reduces the oxygen-carrying capacity of the blood.

Because smoking narrows the size of the arteries, it also causes a ten-fold increased risk of peripheral artery disease as well as a significantly increased risk of abdominal aortic aneurysm. An aneurysm is a bulge in a blood vessel generally caused by a weakening of the arterial wall from atherosclerosis and can be dangerous because it may burst. The aorta, the main artery leading away from the heart, can sometimes develop an aneurysm. Aortic aneurysms usually occur in the abdomen below the kidneys (abdominal aortic aneurysm or AAA). AAA is the thirteenth leading cause of death in the United States and the tenth leading cause of death in men over age 55. Longevity secret? Control diabetes and stop smoking—these are two major risk factors for AAA.

Quitting smoking lowers your risk of heart disease, and the benefits start almost immediately after you quit. Bottom line: if you smoke, partner with your doctor in a structured smoking cessation program. If you are a smoker, quitting smoking is the single most important lifestyle measure you can do to increase your overall longevity.

High Blood Pressure

Of the nearly one in three Americans with high blood pressure (hypertension), one third of them don't know they have it! Thus, high blood pressure is often called the "silent killer."

How do you know if you have high blood pressure? You need to get it measured, and the best place for this is your doctor's office. Home blood pressure monitors, especially the arm cuff ones, may be effective, but if your arm is large or small, the blood pressure cuff may not fit properly and the reading may not be accurate. Also, certain wrist and finger blood pressure machines may not be accurate.

Blood pressure is categorized according to the directive of the Seventh Joint National Committee on Prevention, Detection, Evaluation, and Treatment of High Blood Pressure:

- High blood pressure is a systolic blood pressure (top number in the blood pressure reading) of 140 mmHg or higher or a diastolic blood pressure (lower number in the blood pressure reading) of 90 mmHg or higher.

- Normal blood pressure is a systolic blood pressure of less than 120 mmHg and a diastolic blood pressure of less than 80 mmHg.

- Prehypertension is defined as a systolic blood pressure of 120 to 139 mmHg or a diastolic blood pressure of 80 to 89 mmHg. People with prehypertension are at increased risk of eventually developing hypertension.

If you are diagnosed with high blood pressure, it's important to follow the recommended treatment. This may include diuretics, beta blockers, ACE inhibitors, and calcium channel blockers. (We'll discuss beta blockers and ACE inhibitors later in the chapter.) Exercise, healthy diet, and weight maintenance are also important for maintaining a healthy blood pressure.

> **Doctors' Orders** _____
>
> The Dietary Approaches to Stop Hypertension (DASH) diet is recommended to help control blood pressure. The DASH diet is rich in grains, fruits, vegetables, and low-fat dairy products. It limits fat, saturated fat, and cholesterol and provides plenty of fiber, potassium, calcium, and magnesium. Sodium intake is limited to no more than 2,300 mg a day. A 2005 study showed that reducing some carbohydrates in the DASH diet and replacing them with protein or unsaturated fats may reduce blood pressure further. Protein sources recommended include nuts and seeds, beans, poultry, fish, meat, egg substitutes, fat-free dairy products, and vegetable-based meat substitutes. Sources of unsaturated fats include olive oil, canola oil, avocados, nuts, and seeds.

Don't ignore high blood pressure. It can lead to atherosclerosis, or hardened arteries, which in turn cause a decrease of blood flow to the muscles of the heart. Decreased blood to the heart can lead to angina (chest pain due to a lack of blood carrying oxygen to the heart). It can also lead to a heart attack (caused by a prolonged interruption of blood flow to the heart muscle).

Cholesterol

Cholesterol is a fatty, waxy substance produced naturally in the liver. When we talk about cholesterol levels, we are generally referring to a group of lipids or fats in the bloodstream—the result of how much the liver makes, along with what your diet contributes. It's important to know your cholesterol numbers:

◆ Total cholesterol is the total amount of cholesterol measured in your blood; a normal level is now considered less than 200.

◆ LDL cholesterol is often referred to as the *bad* cholesterol. A good LDL is less than 130; an optimal level is less than 100. The new AHA recommendations include getting your LDL down to 70 for both men and women at high risk for coronary artery disease.

◆ HDL cholesterol is the *good* cholesterol. Men should have a level over 40, and women should be over 50.

◆ Triglycerides, another blood fat that is measured in routine blood tests, should be under 150.

These lipids are affected by many factors, including the foods you eat, your level of activity, your family history, and whether or not you have diabetes. For example, LDL cholesterol tends to go up if you eat a lot of saturated fat, or are sedentary and overweight. Your HDL tends to drop and triglycerides go up if you have diabetes or eat a lot of refined carbohydrates.

High levels of cholesterol lead to a narrowing of the arteries in the body, including those of the heart, which causes heart disease. Over 1 million Americans have high cholesterol and 37 million have a cholesterol level over 240, which is associated with a high risk of heart disease.

The National Cholesterol Education Program recommends a cholesterol check at least every five years. If your cholesterol is high, your doctor may recommend lifestyle changes and put you on a low fat/low cholesterol diet. If your cholesterol remains elevated, and if you have other risk factors for heart disease, you may be advised to start a statin medication, such as Zocor or Lipitor, to lower your cholesterol.

Words to the Wise

Keep these tips in mind:
- ◆ Reducing saturated fat in your diet will lower your LDL cholesterol.
- ◆ Reducing trans fats in your diet will lower your LDL and raise your HDL.
- ◆ Eating healthy oils such as olive oil will lower your LDL and raise your HDL.
- ◆ Eating more fiber will lower your LDL.
- ◆ Eating more fish will lower your triglycerides.
- ◆ Exercising and losing excess weight will lower your LDL and raise your HDL.
- ◆ Drinking alcohol in moderation will raise your HDL. Too much alcohol will raise your triglycerides and is also harmful to the heart muscle.
- ◆ Quitting smoking will raise your HDL.

Diabetes

High blood sugar is toxic to many parts of the body, including the heart, and persistently elevated blood sugar can accelerate heart disease. Diabetes used to be defined as a fasting blood sugar above 140, but adverse effects on the body probably begin with fasting blood sugar levels above 85. A fasting blood sugar between 100 and 125 is defined as prediabetes, or impaired fasting glucose. Many people have prediabetes for years and never know it. Knowing your fasting blood sugar is crucial in maintaining cardiovascular longevity.

Diabetes that occurs in adults is usually type 2 diabetes (also known as adult-onset diabetes), and is invariably associated with being overweight and sedentary. You are at risk for type 2 diabetes if you are over 45, overweight, African American, Latino, Native American, Asian American, or a Pacific Islander, or if you have a family history of diabetes.

To test for type 2 diabetes, get your blood sugar checked. After an overnight fast, your fasting blood sugar should be under 100. If it's between 100 and 125, this is called impaired fasting glucose, or IFG. Your doctor may have you do an oral glucose tolerance test. This test involves drinking a specific amount of a glucose drink, then testing the blood sugar two hours later. A glucose level between 140 and 199 at two hours is considered abnormal. This is also referred to as Impaired Glucose Tolerance, or IGT. Together, IFG and IGT constitute prediabetes and elevate your risk for heart disease, stroke, and dementia. You will read more about diabetes in Chapter 14.

One study of adults aged 40 to 75 found that over 40 percent of them had prediabetes—either IGT, IFT, or both—and most of them didn't know it. Don't wait until you develop frank (actual) diabetes; get your blood sugar checked on a regular basis, especially if you have any risk factors. Type 2 diabetes is largely preventable, *if* you take care of yourself *now*—this means eating a healthy diet, exercising, and maintaining a healthy weight.

Obesity and inactivity are also significant risk factors for the development of coronary artery disease. Thus, if you are obese or have a sedentary lifestyle, it's important to address these factors, as they play a strong role in your heart's longevity. Refer to Chapters 5 and 6 for more on these topics.

Metabolic Syndrome

Metabolic syndrome, or Syndrome X, is a constellation of abnormalities that puts you at much higher risk of heart disease. According to the World Health Organization, you have metabolic syndrome if you have at least three of the following five abnormalities:

- Overweight with truncal obesity (waist circumference over 40 inches in men and over 35 in women)

- Fasting triglycerides over 150

- Low HDL (good) cholesterol (under 40 for men and under 50 for women)

- High blood pressure

- Increased fasting blood glucose (over 100)

If you have three or more of the above, your risk of heart disease is significantly elevated.

Markers of Inflammation

Inflammation is yet another factor that may increase your risk for heart disease Why? Blockages in the blood vessels, including those of the heart, are thought to be accelerated by inflammation present within the body. Cigarette smoking, hypertension, certain types of fats present in the body ("atherogenic lipoproteins"), sedentary lifestyles, and high blood sugar all accelerate this inflammation. These risk factors give rise to the release of various chemicals and the activation of cells involved in the inflammatory process. These lead to *plaque* formation and plaque disruption, including formation of blood clots. These may ultimately lead to heart attacks.

def•i•ni•tion

Plaque is formed from cholesterol, fat, calcium, and other substances in the blood. When blood cholesterol levels are high, there is a greater chance that plaque will build up on the artery walls. This process begins as early as the teenage years and progresses with age.

A heart attack occurs when blood supply to part of the heart muscle is severely reduced or blocked, due to narrowing in one of the coronary arteries. If blood supply is cut off for more than a few minutes, muscle cells in the heart may be permanently injured or die from lack of oxygen.

The high-sensitivity CRP blood test or "hs CRP" measures very mild levels of persistent inflammation in the blood. This inflammation is believed to put you at added risk of heart disease. The Centers for Disease Control recommends that if a person's cardiovascular risk score is low, no test is immediately warranted. If a person is of intermediate risk, the hs CRP can help predict a cardiovascular or stroke event and help point to the need for further evaluation and therapy. A person with a high risk score or established heart disease or stroke should be treated intensively regardless of hs CRP levels.

There are also other tests used to measure inflammation, such as the fibrinogen level, but they are not used as often as the hs CRP.

What can help to reduce inflammation? Once again, exercise, healthy diet, and weight maintenance are the answers! Cholesterol-lowering medications and aspirin may also help reduce inflammation.

Longevity Facts

Don't think you need to go to the dentist? Think again! Untreated gum disease causes inflammation in the gums as well as in the bloodstream, and this inflammation can probably increase your risk of vascular disease. Floss your teeth and fix your heart all in one swipe!

The Stress Factor

Studies have shown that people who have too much stress may be at greater risk of having coronary artery disease. Stress creates certain changes in the body that may predispose to a heart attack, such as speeding up the heart rate, increasing cortisol levels, increasing glucose, increasing blood pressure, and weakening the immune system.

People sometimes respond to stress with unhealthy habits, such as smoking, overeating or eating salty or high-fat foods, and not exercising. It has been definitively shown that people with heart disease are more likely to have a heart attack during times of stress.

Much that causes stress cannot be immediately changed—job stress, financial/marital stressors, or illness. Thus, doctors recommend changing your behavioral response to stress, when the stress cannot be removed. This could include seeking counseling, taking depression and anxiety medications, meditating, seeking spiritual fulfillment, or starting a hobby. These changes may save your life.

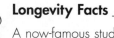

Longevity Facts

A now-famous study done at Case Western Reserve University looked at 10,000 men who had risk factors for heart disease, including high cholesterol, high blood pressure, age over 50, diabetes, and electrocardiogram abnormalities. A question was posed to these men, "Does your wife show you her love?" Surprisingly enough, men who answered "no"—that they did not feel loved—had almost twice as much angina than men who answered "yes." The study came to the conclusion that a wife's love balances out the risk of angina, even in the presence of risk factors.

Dietary Factors

If you want to help ensure a healthy heart, be mindful of incorporating the following elements into your diet:

◆ *Total fat intake:* 25 to 35 percent of dietary calories, most in the form of healthy oils.

◆ *Saturated fat intake:* Less than 7 percent of calories.

◆ *Trans fat intake:* Less than 1 percent of calories.

◆ *Fiber:* 20 to 35 g per day.

◆ *Cholesterol:* Less than 300 mg a day. Less than 200 mg a day if you have high LDL cholesterol.

◆ *Sodium:* 1,500 mg if high risk (HTN, certain ethnicities). Less than 2,300 mg for everyone else.

◆ *Alcohol:* No more than one drink a day for women; no more than two drinks a day for men.

◆ *Fish:* Two times a week. Consider taking daily omega-3 supplements if you've had a heart attack or if you have high triglycerides.

◆ *Fruits and vegetables:* 5 to 10 servings a day.

If you've had a heart attack, the American Heart Association now recommends that you take fish oil every day. Take a total of 1,000 mg of EPA and DHA combined; read the labels to determine how much is in each capsule. Fish oil can also help to lower high blood triglycerides. Much higher levels are needed for this, up to 3,000 to 5,000 mg per day; talk to your doctor first.

Gender Differences in Heart Disease

Women who want to live long and healthy lives should focus first and foremost on preventing heart disease. A 2003 Harris Poll showed a mere 13 percent of women thought heart disease was their biggest health risk. But over 500,000 women will die each year from cardiovascular disease—more than all cancers combined. Or looking at it a different way, 50 percent of all women will die of heart disease or stroke. In fact, since the mid-1980s, more women than men have died every year from heart disease.

There are a few important distinctions in cardiovascular disease in women compared with men:

◆ Low levels of HDL (good cholesterol) and high levels of triglycerides are bigger cardiac risk factors in women than men.

◆ Women are more likely than men to have atypical symptoms of heart disease. Thus, diagnosis of heart disease is more often missed in women. Women are also more likely to get less aggressive treatment once they are diagnosed.

◆ Type 2 diabetes is a stronger contributing risk factor in women than in men for heart disease.

◆ Depression is more common in women than men. And depression increases the risk of heart disease by two to three times, compared with those with similar risk factors who are not depressed.

◆ Angioplasty may not work as well in women as in men.

So what should women do? Stay active, know your risks, know your numbers, keep your weight normal, and partner with your doctor in being aggressive about diagnosing and treating heart disease.

Heart Screenings

You've had some pain in the middle of your chest—you are not having it anymore, but you have a couple of risk factors for heart disease and so you make an appointment with the doctor. What's next? Your doctor may order one of a few types of heart screenings to determine how your heart is functioning. These can include a stress test—of which there are many types—and some imaging studies, as well as more aggressive measures, such as cardiac catheterization.

Stress tests can be life-saving, because they can lead to early detection of heart disease. Almost 50 percent of deaths from heart disease are sudden cardiac death, and many of these cases are in patients who were not diagnosed or were underdiagnosed.

There are various types of stress tests. The simplest is an EKG treadmill test in which you walk on a treadmill at increasing speeds while you are hooked up to an EKG; changes in the tracing of the EKG as you exercise are used to assess the possibility of heart disease.

A stress echocardiogram is similar to a stress EKG, except that an echocardiogram picture of your heart is also obtained, both at rest and during exercise. This allows the cardiologist to assess the global functioning of the heart muscle during exercise; it also provides information about your heart valves as well as the blood flow through the heart.

> ### Doctors' Orders
>
> It is advisable to partner with your physician in making the decision to have a stress test. Some indicators for a stress test may be one or more of the following:
>
> ◆ Evaluation of chest pain
> ◆ Beginning a new exercise program
> ◆ Multiple heart disease risk factors
> ◆ Decreasing exercise tolerance
> ◆ Unexplained shortness of breath or dizziness
> ◆ History of a prior heart attack
> ◆ Genetic predisposition to heart disease

Sometimes a radionucleotide stress test, such as a persantine thallium or a dobutamine thallium test, is ordered. These tests are often used for patients who are unable to exercise on a treadmill because of arthritis or other medical conditions.

Medications That Help Heart Longevity

In the not-too-distant past, the diagnosis of heart disease was a death sentence, but not anymore. In addition to simple aspirin, there are multiple medications used for heart disease that extend both the length and quality of life.

Medications that help your heart live longer are some of the most common heart medications prescribed. Given to the right patient for the right reason, these medications can indeed be lifesavers.

Aspirin

Aspirin prevents blood clots and makes platelets less sticky. It can help to prevent a heart attack from happening in the first place and can also prevent a heart attack from recurring. Because it can also be associated with abnormal bleeding—both in the gastrointestinal tract and in the brain—it is only recommended for those at risk. Talk to your doctor prior to taking routine aspirin.

Statins

These are prescription cholesterol-lowering medications that also stabilize plaque in arteries. They may also have anti-inflammatory effects in the cardiovascular system. These include medications such as Zocor and Lipitor. Multiple studies have shown that statin medications reduce lipid levels and also reduce the risk of heart attack and stroke, especially for people with multiple risk factors.

How low should your cholesterol be? The American Heart Association recommends that the target LDL for those at high risk is 100, and for those at very high risk, the target LDL is 70. Research has shown that lowering mildly elevated cholesterol reduces the risk of heart attack by 24 percent in high-risk patients. Thus, reducing cholesterol, especially if you are high risk, is very important if you wish to live a long life. Partner with your physician in determining if your cholesterol medication is effective for you.

ACE Inhibitors

These remarkable medications have multiple uses. They reduce blood pressure and increase longevity in people with congestive heart failure and kidney disease. They are also recommended in people who have had a heart attack. These medications work by reducing the production of a chemical that constricts blood vessels.

Beta Blockers

Like ACE inhibitors, beta blockers have multiple uses. They are used to treat high blood pressure in people with heart disease. They also prolong life if you have had a heart attack or have heart failure. Receiving a beta blocker during a heart attack can decrease short-term and long-term risk of death by 35 percent. Of these life-saving medications, aspirin is available over the counter, while statins, beta blockers, and ACE inhibitors are available as prescriptions only.

The Least You Need to Know

- ◆ By decreasing your risk of heart disease, you are taking care of the number-one killer of both men and women.

- ◆ Stopping smoking, decreasing cholesterol, managing diabetes, maintaining your weight, and staying physically active are important changes you can make to keep your heart healthy.

◆ Nearly half of all cardiovascular deaths are sudden heart attacks. Know the atypical signs of chest pain and what screenings are appropriate to prevent these attacks.

◆ Women need to be more aware of heart disease, as it may be more subtle in women than men.

◆ If you have heart disease, learn what medications can extend your life.

Chapter 11

Getting the Fighting Edge on Cancer

In This Chapter

- Demystifying cancer
- Assessing your risk for cancer
- Understanding the role of nutrition and exercise
- Food and supplements that fight cancer
- Environmental factors
- Reducing your risk of developing certain cancers

Many cancers may very well be preventable. This is good news, especially when you consider that the number-two cause of death in both men and women in the United States is cancer, affecting over half a million people each year. Learn how to lead a life free from many of the environmental toxins that have the capability of impacting your genes, your organ systems, and ultimately your life span.

What Is Cancer?

Cells in the body are constantly growing, dividing, and also dying. When all is well, these processes are in balance. Every once in a while, however, the process goes awry and cells grow out of control, forming a tumor.

When a tumor is benign, it will not spread to tissues around it or to distant parts of the body and will not necessarily threaten your life. When a tumor is malignant or cancerous, it invades tissues and disrupts the function of the healthy organs around it. Malignant tumors can also spread to other parts of the body. This occurs when some of the malignant cells break away from the original tumor and enter the bloodstream or the lymphatic system where they are then carried to distant parts of the body. This process of distant spread is called *metastasis*. Cancerous tumors will generally cause death, if not removed from the body either by surgery or chemotherapy.

Pinpointing Risk Factors

Risk factors are those things that increase your risk of getting a certain disease, such as cancer and heart disease. Certain risk factors are under your control—nutrition, for example. Others are not.

The greatest risk factors for cancer *not* under your control include your age (the biggest risk factor for many cancers) and your family history. However, most of those factors that can increase your risk of cancer *are* under your control, at least to some extent. These include:

- Nutrition

- Exercise and weight maintenance

- Smoking and exposure to secondhand smoke

- Alcohol

- Sunlight exposure (UV exposure can lead to skin cancers)

- Exposure to certain chemicals, pollutants, viruses, and bacteria

- Exposure to hormones

Longevity Facts

The Centers for Disease Control (CDC) and National Cancer Institute (NCI) report that approximately 30 percent of all cancer deaths are attributable to tobacco use.

Cancer researchers estimate that 80 to 90 percent of cancers are due to these environmental influences, while 30 percent of cancers may be due to poor diet and inadequate exercise. Obesity is fatal when it comes to cancer. A study published in 2003 in the *New England Journal of Medicine* showed a definitive link between obesity and cancer. In the study, 900,000 adults were studied for a period of 16 years. The heaviest adults—those with a body mass index greater than 40—had death rates from all cancers combined that were 52 percent higher (for men) and 62 percent higher (for women) than the rates in men and women of normal weight.

By taking care of yourself and minimizing your exposure to unhealthy habits and toxins, you greatly enhance your ability to fight cancer and increase your longevity.

Knowing Your Family History

Some cancers definitely seem to have a genetic influence, meaning that if family members had those cancers, especially first-degree relatives, then you are at higher risk as well. Does this mean you are going to get that cancer? No! But it does mean that appropriate screening and certain lifestyle measures will ensure that you minimize your risk. The most important inherited cancers include breast, colon, prostate, ovarian, and melanoma skin cancer.

Everyone should get appropriate routine cancer screenings, such as mammography in women and colonoscopy in both men and women. If you feel you are at higher risk of cancer because of your family history, talk to your doctor about prevention and earlier testing, if indicated. Reducing your environmental exposure to toxins such as smoke and other pollutants, eating a healthy diet, and exercising will all help to reduce your likelihood of developing cancer.

Women (and sometimes men) with a very strong family history of breast and/or ovarian cancer are most often referred for genetic testing to look for the two genes that have been most strongly associated with these cancers. These two genes are called BRCA 1 and BRCA 2; these are mutations (alterations) in the DNA that can increase the chance of healthy breast cells becoming malignant.

Women who test positive for BRCA 1 and BRCA 2 are at much higher risk for these cancers, especially before the age of 50. Additionally, they may also be at higher risk of colon cancer.

Breast cancer risk (and possibly prostate cancer risk) is also increased in men with the BRCA 1 or 2 genes (mainly with BRCA 2). Other cancers also occur more frequently in people with BRCA 2, including pancreas, stomach, gallbladder, lymphoma, and melanoma.

What can you do about this? Women who test positive for BRCA 1 or 2 may choose to have their ovary and breast tissue removed, which significantly lowers their risk of cancer and increases their longevity (though it does not completely eliminate the risk).

Preventing Cancer

Many cancers are felt to be preventable if we adhere to a healthy lifestyle that includes proper nutrition, weight maintenance, regular exercise, and avoidance. What better way to prolong your life than to avoid cancer?

Nutrition

While it's difficult to do studies looking at how one particular food ingredient or vitamin might help you prevent cancer and live longer, a number of studies looking at the habits and health outcomes of big groups of people suggest that poor nutritional habits probably account for about 30 percent of all cancers. For example, a high-fat diet is believed to increase your risk of cancer of the colon, prostate, and uterus. People who are obese and inactive have a higher risk of cancer of the breast, colon, uterus, kidney, and esophagus.

Want to increase your longevity? Then pay attention to your diet! Multiple population studies have shown that countries in which people have lower intakes of fat and animal foods and higher intakes of plant foods, including fruits, vegetables, nuts, and legumes, have significantly lower levels of cancer, as well as of heart disease, diabetes, Alzheimer's disease, and high blood pressure. So while you're waiting to see which vitamin is really *the* one that's going to add years to your life, try eating more fruits and veggies and less fat instead. All of the goodness of veggies hasn't been packaged in pill form. Eat your vegetables!

Exercise

Exercise is also important in cancer prevention, probably because it reduces the incidence of obesity. Recent data has suggested that 20 percent of deaths from cancer in women and 14 percent in men are the result of being overweight or obese. Regular exercise is strongly associated with a reduced risk of colon and breast cancer; prostate, lung, ovarian, and endometrial cancers are probably impacted as well. So stay fit, stay aerobic, and stay alive!

Cancer-Fighting Foods and Supplements

Although risk factors such as smoking and obesity probably play a bigger role in cancer prevention than do individual foods, great nutrition is a relatively easy way to incorporate cancer risk reduction into your lifestyle. Specific nutrients may have an impact on a cancer's ability to spread. As you'll see in a moment, certain nutrients can also affect the genes that put you at risk for cancer. Let's review some of the best cancer-fighting foods.

Dark-Colored Fruits and Veggies

Green, red, purple, and blue fruits and veggies—such as spinach, beets, pomegranates, and blueberries—are loaded with nature's antioxidants and anti-inflammatory plant chemicals. These include carotenes and polyphenols, which protect your DNA and reduce your risk of disease.

Doctors' Orders _____

You can have too much of a good thing! Too much beta-carotene from supplements can lead to an 18 percent increase in lung cancer. If taking supplements, take the recommended daily dosage; do not exceed it. There are no studies to suggest that foods high in beta-carotene, such as carrots and sweet potatoes, will increase your risk of lung cancer.

Cruciferous Veggies

These vegetables—which include broccoli, cauliflower, cabbage, and Brussels sprouts— are loaded with several chemicals, including sulphorophane and indole-3-carbinol. Population studies suggest that consumption of these vegetables on a regular basis may reduce the risk of certain cancers.

Vitamin D

While many of us think about vitamin D as the bone vitamin, it actually has many functions, one of which seems to be cancer prevention. Be sure to get at least 800 to

1,000 units per day from a supplement (vitamin D_3, also known as cholecalciferol), especially if you are over 65.

Selenium

Selenium is a mineral that may reduce the ability of cancers to spread; the data seems strongest for prostate cancer. Selenium might also help prevent colon, stomach, and lung cancers. Selenium is toxic if taken in too large amounts. The recommended intake is about 55 mcgm per day and can usually be obtained in a multivitamin.

Folate

Folate, which helps regulate cell division, is one of the B vitamins found in leafy greens and orange juice. Optimum intake of this vitamin may be associated with a reduction in cancer, especially pancreatic cancer and possibly colon and esophageal cancer. Many adults do not get the recommended dose of folate in their food, so consider taking a multivitamin or B-complex tablet to ensure you get an adequate intake. The recommended dose is 400 to 800 mcgm per day.

Flax Seed and Fish Oil

These are both sources of omega-3 fatty acids, although fish oil is a much richer source than flax. Omega-3 fatty acids may help to reduce tumor growth, especially breast and prostate cancer, although data is preliminary in humans.

Tea

Tea contains catechins—powerful antioxidants that are believed to exert protective benefits against cancer. Green tea probably has the highest amount, followed by oolong and black tea. Try drinking 2 to 4 cups a day.

Mushrooms

Mushrooms are a source of protein, fiber, B vitamins, and vitamins C and D. They also contain ergosterol and chitin, which stimulate the immune system; these might help resist tumor growth.

Aspirin

Daily aspirin use may protect against several cancers, including cancers of the colon, esophagus, ovary, breast, and prostate. Aspirin can have serious side effects, however, including bleeding in the stomach and the brain, so talk to your doctor before starting to take it.

Epigenetics

Epigenetics is a fascinating new science that looks at how certain environmental factors, particularly certain chemicals and nutrients, may have an impact on how our genes are switched on and off. For example, certain genes are known to increase our risk of cancer.

Epigenetics is finding that certain protective nutrients in our food can keep these genes turned *off* and prevent them from starting a cancer. These nutrients may also protect us from obesity, diabetes, and heart disease. Conversely, nutritional deficiencies, as well as exposure to certain environmental chemicals, may unmask these cancer genes and allow them to get expressed, resulting in illness.

Most recently, a chemical called bisphenol-A, found in hard plastics such as water bottles and baby bottles, has come under fire for its epigenetic potential to cause harm. When pregnant mice are exposed to this chemical, some of the pups they give birth to are genetically at higher risk of obesity, diabetes, heart disease, and cancer. Also fascinating is the fact that certain nutrients and foods, particularly B vitamins, soy, cruciferous vegetables, and green tea, seem to protect against these changes. This may explain why a healthy diet can help protect us against cancer and obesity. There are still many unanswered questions, but until more is known, pregnant women and young children would be better off avoiding plastics with bisphenol-A.

> **Words to the Wise**
>
> Many cancer researchers estimate that up to 80 percent of cancers are attributable to environmental exposures and lifestyle factors. Foremost of these environmental exposures are tobacco smoke and obesity. This data was reported in the *Journal of the National Cancer Institute* (1981) and in *Recent Results in Cancer Research* (1998).

Tossing the Toxins

There is still much that's unknown about how many of the man-made chemicals in our environment ultimately influence our risk of cancer and our longevity. However, while we wait for more definitive data, it's prudent to minimize your exposure to toxins when you can. Try to do the following, especially if your family history puts you at high personal risk of cancer:

Longevity Facts

You can reduce your intake of pesticides by about 90 percent if you avoid the 12 most commonly contaminated fruits and veggies, also referred to as the "Dirty Dozen": peaches, apples, sweet bell peppers, celery, nectarines, strawberries, cherries, pears, imported grapes, spinach, lettuce, and potatoes. Go for the organic versions of these!

♦ Eat cruciferous vegetables every day for their cancer-fighting chemicals.

♦ Choose dark-colored fruits and veggies loaded with nature's antioxidants.

♦ Eat organic produce when you can.

♦ If you eat meat and other animal foods, consider investing (and yes, it's an investment) in hormone/pesticide/antibiotic-free products that will lessen your exposure to these chemicals.

♦ Avoid grilling meat and cooking foods at high temperatures to minimize your intake of HCAs and those polycyclic aromatic hydrocarbons. (See "Chemicals in Our Foods" later in this chapter.)

♦ Avoid Teflon cookware, if possible; try cast-iron products instead, which are safer and also provide dietary iron for you, to boot.

♦ Avoid using plastic water bottles and plastic products for infants and young children; avoid heating food in plastic containers in the microwave.

♦ Consider using chemical-free cosmetics when you can.

♦ Stay away from other obvious toxins—tobacco, alcohol, pollutants, and industrial chemicals.

Reducing Your Risk of Cancer

Except perhaps in the case of lung cancer, where tobacco is the main culprit, many cancers have multiple factors that play a role in their onset. By being aware of your risk factors, practicing good health habits—which includes regular exams—and doing all in your power to eliminate environmental toxins and negative lifestyle habits, you will be doing your part to reduce your chances of developing certain cancers.

Lung

Lung cancer is mostly seen in folks who are exposed to tobacco products. Beta-carotene supplements have also been linked to an increased risk of lung cancer, although foods high in carotenes are protective. Preliminary data also suggests a higher risk in those people who eat a lot of red and processed meats.

Want to reduce your risk of lung cancer? Eat fruits and veggies high in carotenes (such as sweet potatoes) and selenium (such as Brazil nuts), and get in your daily exercise, which has also been shown to be protective.

Colorectal Cancer (CRC)

Risk of this cancer is increased by meat consumption (especially red and processed meats), alcohol, and obesity.

Reduce your risk of colon cancer by exercising and staying lean. Other things that may reduce your risk include calcium supplements, selenium, folic acid, fruits and veggies, and dietary fiber. Polyp removal via colonoscopy may also reduce CRC.

Breast

Reduce your risk of breast cancer by staying active and avoiding obesity, especially if you are past menopause. Obesity after menopause increases the risk by almost three-fold for the heaviest women. Breast feeding also reduces the risk.

Several prescription drugs, including Tamoxifen and Evista, reduce your risk, though Tamoxifen may increase the risk of uterine cancer. Adequate vitamin D intake may help to reduce the risk.

> **Doctors' Orders**
>
> The use of estrogen and progesterone together for menopausal women can reduce the risk of colon cancer by 20 to 40 percent, but it also raises the risk of breast cancer and vascular disease. If using these hormones, talk with your doctor to inform yourself of the risks and benefits.

Breast cancer risk is increased by alcohol consumption and by the use of estrogen and progesterone after menopause.

Some, but not all, studies have suggested that exposure to organochlorine pesticides, such as DDT and PCPs, can also increase breast cancer risk.

Cervical

If you are a teenage or young adult woman, you can reduce your risk of this cancer by getting the new HPV vaccine. This protects against the sexually transmitted human papilloma virus, the virus that causes most cases of cervical cancer. Regular pap smears may decrease mortality from cervical cancer by more than 80 percent.

Women who are infected with HPV and who also smoke have two to three times the risk of cervical cancer as women with HPV who don't smoke.

Ovarian

The easiest way to prevent ovarian cancer and increase your longevity is to use combination oral contraceptives (estrogen + progesterone). Pre-menopausal women who use this type of birth control pill may reduce their risk of ovarian cancer by up to 80 percent.

Doctors' Orders _____

Oral contraceptives may have side effects, including increased risk of blood clots. They may also cause a very slight increase in breast cancer, but this risk stops as soon as you stop taking the pill. Talk to your doctor to see if oral contraceptives are appropriate for you.

Uterine

Birth control pills reduce the risk of uterine cancer. This risk is reduced by 50 percent after only 4 years of continuous use, and up to 72 percent after 12 or more years of use. Women who use estrogen therapy after menopause, and who still have their uterus, must take progesterone with their estrogen in order to decrease their risk of developing uterine cancer.

Obesity and alcohol are also associated with a higher risk of uterine cancer.

Prostate

For men interested in keeping their prostate healthy, the most recent evidence shows that foods containing lycopene (especially cooked tomato products) and selenium or a selenium supplement (100 to 200 mcgm per day) are protective.

Vitamin E, beans, and other legumes may also help. The medication Finasteride has been shown to reduce the incidence of prostate cancer but has not yet been proven to prolong life. One recent study looked at adding flax seed meal to the diets of men with prostate cancer before they went in for surgery. Those men taking 30 g of flax seed meal per day for three weeks prior to having their prostates removed showed a significant reduction in tumor growth.

There is some evidence that diets high in processed meats such as bacon and salami may increase prostate cancer risk.

Skin

You already know about the importance of sunscreens and sunblocks to help prevent skin cancer. And while this makes good intuitive sense, there actually is not a lot of good data to show that these products actually prevent skin cancer, including melanoma. We do know, however, that people who have high sun exposure—in countries such as Australia, for example—also have very high rates of skin cancer. Bottom line? Use your sunblock just to be sure, and stay out of the sun during the hottest times of the day.

Esophageal

The best way to prevent this cancer is to avoid tobacco, alcohol abuse, and obesity. A high intake of fruits and veggies, especially those containing beta-carotene and vitamin C, may also help. Limiting your intake of fresh and processed meats may also reduce your risk.

Tobacco in all forms is carcinogenic (cigarettes, chewing tobacco, etc.). Smoking alone is a big risk factor for these cancers; if you add alcohol abuse to the mix, the risk of esophageal cancer goes up two to seven times.

Stomach

Fruits, veggies, and produce from the onion family all seem to protect against stomach cancer. Foods high in selenium may also help.

High salt intake seems to increase the risk of stomach cancer. Some experts now recommend limiting sodium for most people to under 1,500 mg per day. High intakes of processed meats may also increase risk. Infection with the bacteria *Helicobacter pylori*, which is associated with stomach ulcers, can also increase the risk of stomach cancer. This infection can be diagnosed with either a blood test or a culture taken from the stomach by a gastroenterologist.

Identifying Harmful Habits

Cancer specialists estimate that our environment and our personal health habits, in particular—including tobacco and alcohol use, poor nutrition, and obesity—cause the vast majority of cancers. This is where the element of personal control enters the picture and where you can have the greatest impact on enhancing your life span and your health span.

Tobacco

Tobacco reduces longevity more than just about anything else in our environment. According to the National Cancer Institute, tobacco is responsible for more than 180,000 deaths every year in the United States. Smokers are at higher risk of cancer of the mouth, vocal cords, throat, esophagus, lung, stomach, pancreas, bladder, kidney, cervix, and blood cells (leukemia).

People who are exposed to secondhand smoke are also at risk for these cancers, though not to the same extent as people who smoke. People who use chewing tobacco or snuff are at higher risk of cancer of the mouth.

Quitting smoking results in immediate benefits. It is estimated that quitting will increase your life span anywhere from 3 to 10 years. If it's hard to quit on your own, talk to your doctor about medications to help you kick the habit.

Alcohol

Excess alcohol (more than two drinks per day) intake over many years increases the risk of many cancers, including cancer of the breast, uterus, mouth, throat, esophagus, liver, and colon; lung and pancreatic cancer may be increased as well. The more you drink, the higher your risk.

If you also smoke cigarettes, your risk of these cancers is even higher. What's a reasonable person to do? In order to reduce your personal risk of cancer, the American

Cancer Society recommends that women consume one drink per day or less; men should limit their intake to two drinks per day or less. If you already have one of these cancers, or are at high risk for them, you would be better off not drinking at all.

Looking at Hormones

When the Women's Hormone Initiative study results were published in 2001 and showed that *post-menopausal* use of estrogen and progesterone definitely increased a woman's risk of breast cancer, many women in the United States stopped taking these hormones. Recently, a significant drop in breast cancer was noted, believed to be due to this drop in estrogen use.

While hormone use may have its benefits, estrogen, progesterone, testosterone, and other hormones such as DHEA and growth hormone may all be associated with an increased risk of cancer, especially hormonally affected cancers—breast, prostate, ovarian, and uterine cancer. Avoiding *post-menopausal* hormone use, when possible, is the best way to minimize this cancer risk. (Note that *pre-menopausal* use of oral contraceptives is protective against both uterine and ovarian cancer, but may increase the risk of breast cancer.) Other than hormones, chemotherapy drugs used to treat cancer may also increase the risk of other cancers in the future.

Chemical Soup

Every year, Americans are exposed to over 100,000 chemicals that are used in household cleaners, food additives, food production, cosmetics, pesticides, and yard-care products. More are added to the arsenal every year, and many have not been proven to be safe. In addition, sometimes the way we prepare foods can cause toxic changes that are carcinogenic. Most of the time safe alternatives are available. Here's the rundown on what these chemicals are and how you can avoid them.

Chemicals in Our Foods

Acrylamide is a carcinogenic chemical that can form in some foods that are heated to high temperatures; relatively high levels are found in potato chips and french fries. In 2002, the World Health Organization concluded that acrylamide was probably a major health concern for humans. More research is underway.

Heterocyclic amines (HCAs) are carcinogenic chemicals that develop in meat, poultry, or fish when cooked at high temperatures.

Polycyclic aromatic hydrocarbons are carcinogens formed when fat from grilled animal foods drips onto the coals; these chemicals can then splash back up and onto your grilled feast. Exposure to these toxins is reduced if you use lower-fat cuts of meat.

Perfluorooctanoic acid (PFOA) is used to make the nonstick coating of Teflon products. This carcinogenic chemical can be released into your cooked food if the pan becomes super hot (over 600 degrees).

Cosmetics and Such

Phthalates are chemicals used to make plastic products softer and more pliable. They are widely used in many products used by consumers: medical equipment, toys, and cosmetics. They are carcinogenic in animals and are also felt to exert hormonal changes in human tissue. They are now banned in the United States in infant toys, bottles, and nipples.

Parabens, a preservative used in deodorants and antiperspirants, acts like an estrogen in the body. Some scientists are concerned that parabens might increase the risk of breast cancer.

Industry

Industrial chemical exposures that can increase your risk of cancer include formaldehyde (used in the medical and funeral industries), vinyl chloride and acrylonitrile (used in the plastics industry), asbestos, benzene, mercury, cadmium, nickel, and PCBs. People exposed to these chemicals in the workplace have a higher risk of cancer, especially brain cancer. Pesticides may exert a hormonal-like effect on tissues and possibly increase the risk of cancer as well.

Radiation exposure is another cancer risk, especially radiation from the nuclear industry, medical x-rays, cosmic rays, and environmental radon. Although cell phones do emit a small amount of radiation, multiple studies have *not* shown an association between their use and brain cancer; however, long-term studies lasting more than 10 years are not yet available.

Bottom line? Increase your longevity by limiting your exposure to toxins whenever possible.

Linking Viruses and Bacteria to Cancers

Certain viral and bacterial infections can increase the risk of cancer. Fortunately, there are vaccinations to protect against some of these:

- *Human papilloma virus (HPV):* Certain strains of this virus are associated with cervical cancer and possibly other cancers as well. There is now a vaccine to protect against most of the strains that do cause cervical cancer.

- *Hepatitis B and C:* Many people who are exposed to the hepatitis B virus recover completely; some, however, will end up with persistent infection which puts them at risk for liver cancer. Hepatitis C is much more likely than hepatitis B to become a chronic infection, and in these people there is a significant risk of cirrhosis and liver cancer. A vaccination is available to prevent hepatitis B infection, but not C.

- *Epstein-Barr virus (EBV):* This virus, which causes mononucleosis, may be associated with a higher risk of rare types of lymphoma.

- *Human immunodeficiency virus (HIV):* Infection with the HIV virus increases one's risk of both lymphoma and Kaposi's sarcoma. No vaccine is yet available; practice safe sex!

- *Helicobacter pylori:* This bacteria, which causes one of the most widespread infections in the world, settles into the stomach lining. It is associated with stomach ulcers but if left untreated is also associated with stomach cancer, as well as lymphoma of the lining of the stomach. The cure rate is high with appropriate antibiotics, although it is not yet certain that eradication of this bacteria definitely reduces the risk of cancer.

Stop Stressing Out

Does stress cause cancer? This is a question many scientists have grappled with. We know that chronic stress can dampen our immune systems and may make us more vulnerable to illnesses, such as the common cold. But can stress cause something more serious, such as cancer?

Some data suggest that people who have experienced the recent death of a spouse or other significant loved one are themselves at higher risk of dying. A number of more recent studies looking at the amount of stress in one's life prior to a diagnosis of cancer, however, have *not* shown a link between stress and the onset of cancer. In fact, some lab animals bred to have no immune systems do not have an increase in most cancers.

More recent intriguing data has suggested, instead, that cancer cells may secrete substances that prevent our healthy immune cells from destroying the cancerous ones. Scientists are now testing, in animals, substances that stimulate the immune cells to make them recognize and destroy the cancer cells. The results are promising, but these treatments are not yet available in humans.

What about stress reduction *after* you've been diagnosed with cancer? Is that likely to help you heal from cancer or live longer? Intriguing research from Dr. David Spiegel at Stanford in the 1980s suggested that support groups helped women with metastatic breast cancer to live longer, but that data has now been questioned. We do know, however, that stress reduction techniques, including meditation, can reduce the anxiety and fear associated with cancer. This can improve the quality of life, even if it does not increase length of life.

The Least You Need to Know

- Many cancers are preventable, with avoidance of toxins and maintenance of a healthy lifestyle.

- Know your family history and your personal risk factors for cancer; talk to your doctor about appropriate screenings.

- Get appropriate vaccinations.

- Avoid exposure to food additives and environmental toxins whenever possible.

- Eat a diet low in animal fat and high in produce and whole grains whenever possible. If you can, go organic.

Chapter 12

Vital Lungs

In This Chapter

◆ The breath of life

◆ Smoking: public enemy number one

◆ You *can* quit!

◆ Environmental detective

◆ Chronic lung disease and longevity

◆ Avoiding respiratory illness

There's a great deal we take for granted with the human body, and it does its best to serve us well. Breathing comes naturally, and we take our lungs for granted. More than 35 million Americans, however, are living with chronic lung disease and the debilitation it causes. The Centers for Disease Control (CDC) estimates that every year, almost 350,000 Americans die of lung disease, making this America's number-three killer, responsible for one in seven of all deaths. Taking care of your lungs is essential to maximize both your health span and your life span.

Healthy Lungs

The lungs are two spongy organs covered by a membrane (the pleura). At their most fundamental level, your lungs function to give oxygen to your body. Every day, your lungs bring in about 8,000 liters of oxygen-rich air to your body, remove waste, and provide a defense from toxins they encounter—dust, pollen, toxic chemicals and airborne pollutants, bacteria, and viruses.

When you inhale, air is carried through the windpipe, or trachea, to your lungs through two major airways called bronchi. Inside the lungs, the bronchi subdivide nearly 20 times into a million smaller airways called bronchioles, which finally end in clusters of tiny air sacs called alveoli, whose job it is to get oxygen into your body and bloodstream.

You can do a great deal to keep your lungs in top working order. Lung tissue becomes scarred with repeated exposure to cigarette smoke and certain environmental pollutants. Avoiding those pollutants, along with quitting the nicotine habit, are two important actions you can take to improve lung function. Also, if you do suffer from specific lung conditions, such as asthma or emphysema, be sure to follow your doctor's instructions for taking care of yourself. Each breath is precious.

Words to the Wise
Exercise to quit smoking! A study published in the June 1999 issue of *Archives of Internal Medicine* of almost 300 women showed that women who exercised regularly while trying to quit smoking were two times as likely to successfully quit smoking. Furthermore, they only gained half the weight as compared to women who quit but did not exercise.

Smoking and Your Health

The best way to keep the alveoli and bronchioles of the lungs in prime working order is to not scar and damage them with cigarette smoke. Smoking doesn't just harm the lungs; it adversely impacts nearly every organ in the body. Smoking is an equal-opportunity health destroyer.

It's Never Too Late to Quit

Smoking causes 438,000 premature deaths a year. That's the bad news. The good news is that smoking's harmful effects can be reversed by quitting smoking. People who quit smoking at age 50 decrease their risk of dying prematurely by 50 percent, compared to those who continue to smoke. And it is never too late—studies have shown that people who quit smoking at age 60 live longer than those who don't quit. If you are a smoker, the healthiest thing you can to increase your longevity is to quit smoking.

The hard part is quitting smoking effectively. Many people who eventually are successful in quitting have tried to quit numerous times before. Don't give up. If you can't do it on your own, partner with your doctor in setting up a structured quit-smoking program. This may include support classes, the nicotine patch, and/or prescription medications.

Longevity Facts

According to the CDC, smoking causes ...

◆ Over 80 percent of lung cancer deaths in men and women.

◆ Cancers of the bladder, oral cavity, pharynx, larynx, esophagus, cervix, kidney, lung, pancreas, and stomach.

◆ Acute myeloid leukemia.

◆ Two to four times greater risk of coronary artery disease, as compared to nonsmokers.

◆ Double the risk of stroke, compared to nonsmokers.

◆ Ten times the risk of narrowing of peripheral arteries.

◆ Abdominal aortic aneurysm.

◆ Lower bone density and increased risk of hip fracture in women.

◆ Ten times increased risk of dying from emphysema.

Nicotine Replacement Products

Nicotine is the chemical in cigarettes that causes the addiction. Smoking cessation remedies include nicotine replacement, which prevents the body from going into physical withdrawal from nicotine and makes quitting more likely to be permanent. Nicotine replacement can come in many forms, including patches, gums, and inhalers. Following is a breakdown of the nicotine replacement products available on the market.

◆ *Nicotine patch:* This is available over the counter and is applied daily, as a part of an eight-week program to quit smoking. The nicotine is absorbed gradually through the skin and reduces the cravings for cigarettes. The dose is gradually tapered over the treatment period. Some people may develop a rash or skin sensitivity to the patch.

◆ *Nicotine gum:* This is available over the counter in 2 and 4 milligram (mg) strengths. The chemical is absorbed through the lining of the mouth. The gum may need to be chewed every one to two hours to release a steady amount of nicotine into the system. The nicotine gum may not be good for people with jaw or dental problems. A nicotine lozenge is also available.

◆ *Nicotine nasal sprays:* These are prescription items that deliver nicotine thorough the lining of the nasal passages. Nicotine is absorbed rapidly with this method of delivery. This may not work for people with sinus problems, such as allergies.

◆ *Nicotine inhaler:* This is also a prescription. The nicotine in the nicotine inhaler is absorbed by the mucous membrane lining in the mouth and throat. The inhaler does *not* deliver the nicotine to the lungs.

Doctors' Orders

The CDC offers the following guidelines for quitting smoking:

◆ Don't smoke any number or any kind of cigarettes. The best option is not to smoke at all. Low tar or "just a few" cigarettes a day still cause lasting damage to the lungs.

◆ Write down why you want to quit. This will help you in outlining your motivations and keep you on track in quitting.

◆ Know that it will take effort to quit smoking. All smokers have signs of nicotine withdrawal; being prepared for this will help you quit effectively.

◆ Stay motivated. Half of all adult smokers have quit, so you can, too.

◆ Get help if you need it.

Other Medications

Buproprion is an antidepressant approved by the FDA in 1997 for help in treating nicotine addiction. Buproprion reduces nicotine withdrawal symptoms and can reduce the urge to smoke. This medication is generally started a couple weeks before you quit smoking and can be effectively used along with nicotine replacement products. Buproprion is contraindicated in people with seizure disorders or eating disorders.

The second drug to be recently approved by the FDA for assistance in smoking cessation is Varenicline, or Chantix. This medication works by easing nicotine withdrawal symptoms and blocking the effects of nicotine in people who resume smoking.

Both Buproprion and Varenicline are prescription medications and need to be obtained from your doctor.

Acupuncture

Many people use acupuncture as an adjunct to quitting smoking. Studies on this method, however, are not that favorable in terms of its effectiveness. The same is true for acupressure, laser therapy, and electrostimulation—not much data supports their use as effective interventions in smoking cessation.

Hypnosis

Hypnosis appears to have better results than quitting cold turkey in helping people—especially men—quit smoking. A study of over 5,000 smokers found that about 30 percent of men and 23 percent of women who used a hypnosis-based treatment were able to quit. Most effective hypnosis treatments are multiple sessions and work best when combined with other smoking cessation interventions.

Environmental Factors in Lung Disease

You can, in large part, control your environment and minimize your exposure to indoor and outdoor air pollutants. The air you breathe impacts both your lungs and your breathing and can lead to chronic diseases. Avoid these chronic respiratory problems by paying attention to your surroundings.

Secondhand Smoke

Secondhand smoke exposure has been shown to increase health risks. Tobacco smoke carries numerous toxic chemicals—at least 250 known to harm humans, and 50 of them known to cause cancer. When you inhale secondhand smoke, you are exposing your body to all these toxins. These harmful chemicals include:

♦ *Hydrogen cyanide:* Used to make chemical weapons

♦ *Formaldehyde:* Used in embalming fluid

- *Ammonia:* A toxic household cleaner

- *Toluene:* A paint thinner

- *Arsenic:* A heavy metal poison

- *Beryllium:* A chemical used to make batteries

- *Vinyl chloride:* Used in the manufacture of plastics

Avoiding secondhand smoke entirely is essential to your health and longevity, so if you live or work in the company of smokers, stay away from their smoke. You will help your body stay healthy.

Environmental Pollutants

Our environment is becoming increasingly polluted, indoors as well as outdoors. Outdoor pollutants include noxious fumes, such as exhaust fumes from cars, chemical fumes, paint fumes, and gasoline fumes. Keep an eye out for high-ozone days and try to say inside when levels are high.

Indoor pollution can be caused by a number of sources, including tobacco smoke, dust, dirt, household chemicals, fireplaces, asbestos, radon, mold and mildew, and animal dander. Indoor pollutants can cause or aggravate asthma and other lung problems and lead to coughs, allergies, and an increased tendency to catch respiratory infections. Indoor pollutants radon and asbestos can lead to cancer. Doctors are now seeing the adverse health effects caused by pollutants in an increased number of asthma cases, compared to just 20 or 30 years ago.

Radon

One of these indoor pollutants, radon, merits some discussion. Radon is an invisible, odorless, tasteless gas which is the second overall leading cause of lung cancer. It is the number-one cause of lung cancer among nonsmokers. Each year, radon kills thousands of Americans and is responsible for 15 percent of lung cancers worldwide. It is classified as a "complete carcinogen" and a "Class A" carcinogen—this is because it can act alone to initiate, promote, and propagate cancer.

To avoid this preventable exposure and its potential health effects, have your home tested for radon. This can be done through a do-it-yourself test, or you can hire a reputable company to do the radon test.

How does radon damage the lungs and cause cancer? Radon enters the lungs through the respiratory tract by riding on smoke and dust particles in the air. These particles then lodge themselves in crevices deep within the lungs, where they penetrate the epithelial cells that line the airways. In some cases, the radon becomes concentrated in areas of the lungs, causing irreversible damage. Once inside the cells, the radon can alter the genetic makeup of the cells, causing cancerous tumors to form.

Chronic Lung Conditions

Certain lung conditions decrease quality of life, in addition to shortening life span. Living with chronic disease, especially chronic lung disease, requires that you follow your doctors' recommendations, take the required medications, and make the recommended lifestyle changes.

Emphysema/COPD

Healthy lungs are like fresh balloons, rhythmically inflating and deflating with ease. Lungs afflicted with emphysema can be likened to floppy balloons, where the air flow is somewhat blocked, and all the air that goes in does not exit out. Five out of six cases of emphysema, or chronic obstructive pulmonary disease (COPD), are a direct result of chronic smoking.

Chronic smoking leads to irreversible changes and scarring of the lungs—this is COPD. This damage then leads to loss of elasticity in the lungs. There is also increased inflammation, thickening, and increased mucous production of the lungs. All of these changes lead to weaker lungs with poor oxygenation.

COPD kills 120,000 people yearly. Approximately 12 million Americans are diagnosed with COPD, and it is estimated that another 12 million have it and don't know it. COPD generally occurs in smokers over the age of 40, and the symptoms can be gradual and slowly progressive.

The symptoms of COPD can include the following:

- Chronic coughing (i.e., the smoker's cough)
- Shortness of breath with activities
- Excessive sputum or phlegm production
- Wheezing

♦ Dyspnea—a feeling that you can't breathe

♦ An increased tendency to catch lung infections

If you are a smoker or a former smoker and are having any of these symptoms, consult with your doctor to see if you have undiagnosed COPD. You can add years to your life by treating this condition early and appropriately.

Asthma

Asthma affects over 15 million adults in the United States and is the reason for more than 13 million office visits yearly to the doctor. The latest studies show that asthma is underdiagnosed and undertreated in the United States.

The *Journal of Allergy and Clinical Immunology* recently published the Real-World Evaluation of Asthma Control and Treatment study (REACT study), which looked at over 1,500 adults with moderate-to-severe asthma. The study found that over 55 percent of the adults with asthma polled had uncontrolled asthma—in spite of the fact they had regular access to health care and were on asthma medications.

To be proactive in treating asthma, physicians recommend the following:

♦ Look for conditions that could be triggering your asthma. These include allergic rhinitis, gastroesphageal reflux, and certain medications. (Aspirin, NSAIDs, and beta blockers can cause asthma.)

♦ Stop smoking and avoid exposure to secondhand smoke.

♦ If you have chronic allergies, get tested for indoor triggers, such as house dust mite, cockroach, and cat and dog allergens.

♦ Keep track of your symptoms, take your medications as prescribed, and follow up with your doctor regularly.

♦ Avoid exposure to unnecessary chemicals, dyes, fragrances, sprays, or vapors.

♦ Allergy-proof your house. This includes minimizing pet dander, cleaning air vents, keeping the humidity below 50 percent, clearing out cockroaches, keeping the house mold-free, and avoiding indoor pollutants, such as wood-burning stoves or unvented stoves.

> **Doctors' Orders**
>
> Be aware of the symptoms of asthma. They can include audible wheezing, coughing, tightness in the chest, and shortness of breath. More severe asthma may show up as difficulty talking, exercising, or walking; severe coughing; shallow and fast breathing; or breathing that is slower than usual.

◆ If you have seasonal allergies that worsen your asthma, get allergy testing and consider allergy shots.

Natural remedies have had some success in treating asthma. Here are some to consider:

◆ Reduce foods that contain arachidonic acid from your diet. These include foods such as egg yolk, shellfish, and meat. It is thought that arachidonic acid increases inflammation and worsens asthma.

◆ Replace the bad (saturated/animal) fats with omega-3 fatty acids—these can reduce the level of arachidonic acid in the body.

◆ Try the herb Butterbur, which has been shown to reduce the number, duration, and severity of asthma attacks. Butterbur, a perennial shrub, contains petasin and isopetasin, which are believed to reduce smooth-muscle spasm and have an anti-inflammatory effect.

◆ Eat a diet rich in fruits and vegetables, including tomatoes, leafy vegetables, and carrots; this may even reduce the incidence of asthma.

◆ Increase your dietary intake of fruit, vitamin C, and manganese; this may reduce asthma symptoms, according to a 2006 study conducted by the University of Cambridge.

Pneumonia, Influenza, and Other Lung Infections

Pneumonia and influenza (the flu) are the seventh leading causes of mortality in the United States, and while these are essentially manageable and reversible infections, over 60,000 people die from them each year. Your best bet to keep from becoming a statistic is to avoid these diseases in the first place. And if you do contract one of them, seeking a physician at the first sign of symptoms is key to avoiding complications.

Doctors' Orders

A small study appearing in the *American Journal of Clinical Nutrition* (2004) showed that only 29 percent of those people who took zinc every day got a cold, flu, or other infection, compared with 88 percent of those taking a placebo. Look for a multivitamin that has 15 to 20 mg of zinc. And here's a supplemental recommendation: exercise! A study reported in the November 2006 issue of *American Journal of Medicine* showed that sedentary post-menopausal women had twice the risk of getting sick compared to women who exercised regularly.

Keeping Germs Away

Wash your hands frequently, especially during the cold and flu season. When you touch something other people have touched and then touch your face (eyes, nose, or mouth), you run the risk of catching whatever disease is making the rounds. Door-knobs, ATM machines, countertops, and computer keyboards can all carry germs. When you wash your hands, use soap and warm water, work up a good lather, and wash for 30 seconds, or about as long as it takes to say the alphabet.

Alcohol-containing hand sanitizers are now preferred in many hospitals and medical settings because they do an excellent job disinfecting the skin. Be sure to get a product that has at least 60 percent alcohol—lower concentrations may not be effective.

Avoid crowds if you can, and avoid people who are sick. If your friend or family member has a cold or the flu, don't get too close. Avoid airplanes or enclosed spaces with crowds during cold and flu season.

Flu and Pneumonia Vaccines

Most people over 65, and those younger with lung conditions or immunocompromised states, such as diabetes or cancer, should get a flu shot each year in the fall. This group should also get a pneumonia vaccine every five to seven years. These two vaccinations can greatly reduce your risk of contracting the flu or pneumonia.

Doctors' Orders _____

Focus on your longevity by ensuring you do not get sick or die from a preventable infection. The CDC recommends flu shots for people who …

◆ Are 50 years of age and older. Because nearly one third of people in this age category in the United States have one or more medical conditions that place them at increased risk for serious flu complications, vaccination is recommended for all people aged 50 and older.

◆ Live in nursing homes and other long-term care facilities that house those with long-term illnesses.

◆ Have any condition that can compromise respiratory function.

◆ Have a weakened immune system.

There are two types of vaccines for the flu, and for those over 50, the recommended choice is the flu shot. The flu shot is an inactivated vaccine (containing killed virus) and is approved for use in people older than six months, including healthy people and people with chronic medical conditions. The nasal-spray flu vaccine is a vaccine made with live, weakened flu viruses that do not cause the flu. The nasal-spray flu vaccine is approved for use in healthy people 2 to 49 years of age who are not pregnant.

Each vaccine contains three influenza viruses: one A (H3N2) virus, one A (H1N1) virus, and one B virus. The viruses in the vaccine change each year, based upon scientists' estimations about which types and strains of viruses will be present that year. It takes two weeks after vaccination for your body to develop antibodies that provide protection against influenza virus infection.

The pneumovax (pneumococcal polysaccharide vaccine) is part of the routine adult *immunization* schedule and should be given to adults over 65 years of age. Many adults who should receive the vaccine don't get it. If you want to prevent your chance of getting pneumonia and are over 65 or have a lung condition, talk to your doctor about getting the pneumonia shot.

def•i•ni•tion

> **Immunizations** are injections given to trigger the immune system to be able to recognize and attack future disease. If you are exposed to the full-blown disease later in life, you will either not become infected or have a much less serious infection.

In 2004, influenza and pneumonia combined were ranked as the eighth leading cause of death in the United States and the sixth leading cause in people over 65. Anywhere from 10 to 20 percent of the U.S. population gets sick with influenza (flu) each year and approximately 226,000 people in the United States are hospitalized with complications from influenza. An average of 36,000 die from the virus and its complications every year. Statistics further show that about 90 percent of deaths due to influenza and pneumonia occur in people aged 65 and over.

It is recommended that you receive the pneumococcal vaccine if you …

◆ Are 65 years old or older.

◆ Have a serious long-term health problem such as heart disease, sickle cell disease, alcoholism, lung disease (not including asthma), diabetes, or liver cirrhosis.

◆ Have a weakened immune system (this could be due to Hodgkin's disease; multiple myeloma; cancer treatment with x-rays or drugs; treatment with long-term steroids; bone marrow or organ transplant; kidney failure; HIV/AIDS; lymphoma, leukemia, or other cancers; nephrotic syndrome; damaged spleen or no spleen).

◆ Are an Alaskan native or from certain Native American populations.

Knowing all this, only 65.7 percent of American adults aged 65 years or older were immunized for influenza and only 65.9 percent for pneumonia. This leaves over 35 percent of the population that could potentially still be vaccinated and avoid these deadly infectious lung diseases.

The longevity take-home here? It just makes sense that all people age 65 and over get vaccinated for the flu and pneumonia, thus decreasing their chances of dying from these infections.

Danger Signs of Respiratory Infections

The way to a long life is to prevent illness. Because pneumonia and influenza are potentially serious diseases, it just makes sense to be able to recognize their symptoms. So how do you know if you have a cold or something more severe, such as pneumonia or influenza? See your doctor if you have any of the following symptoms associated with your respiratory infection:

◆ Persistent cough

◆ Temperature higher than 102°F for two or more days

◆ Chills and sweats

◆ Bloody sputum

◆ Shortness of breath

◆ Increasing weakness or exercise intolerance

◆ Chest pain with breathing

◆ A cold or flu that suddenly takes a turn for the worse

Treating these symptoms aggressively and early may very well save your life.

The Least You Need to Know

◆ Smoking is the leading cause of preventable death in the country.

◆ Quitting smoking can be helped by using nicotine patches and the prescription medications Buproprion and Varenicline.

◆ Emphysema is a significant cause of death and illness in the United States.

◆ Avoid secondhand smoke and environmental pollutants.

◆ If you have asthma, keep it well treated.

◆ Be up-to-date on your flu shots and pneumonia shots.

Chapter 3

Keeping Your Brain Healthy

In This Chapter

- ◆ Your brain as you age
- ◆ Stroke and Alzheimer's disease
- ◆ Assessing your risk for stroke and dementia
- ◆ Keeping your brain healthy
- ◆ Preventive measures for dementia
- ◆ Important screenings

Healthy lifestyle habits are powerful allies in the fight against debilitating diseases of the brain, slowing—and in some cases, warding off—stroke and Alzheimer's disease. Both of these diseases, as well as other forms of dementia, cause a substantial amount of disability. Recent evidence suggests that many cases of dementia are due to vascular disease in the brain, the same type of process that leads to heart attacks. Fascinating research is also showing that certain supplements and dietary interventions may also help prevent certain brain diseases.

Taking Control of Your Brain's Longevity

There are certain changes that happen to the brain as we age. These include loss of brain mass, decrease in white matter, a decrease in outer surface of the brain, and a decrease in chemical messengers in the brain. This leads to a decrease in brain weight and brain volume. However, scientists have recently discovered that contrary to popular belief, we continue to form new neurons in the mature adult brain as we age.

A decline in brain functioning used to be thought to be due to degenerative changes in the brain called neurofibrillary tangles and senile plaque. However, in a recent study reported in the *Journal of Neurophysiology*, researchers conducted postmortem examinations on the brains of elderly people who had been fully functioning until death. Their brains, surprisingly, had the changes of Alzheimer's disease, with a large amount of plaque and tangles, but none of these patients had any symptoms of Alzheimer's disease. Scientists are now investigating other causes for the deterioration of brain function, including the formation of amyloid deposits in the brain, a process thought to be accelerated by inflammation in the body.

Even though physical changes in the brain occur with Alzheimer's disease, there is an unknown factor. Some people with the changes will get the disease and some will not. This is powerful information, as we do know there are some lifestyle changes we can make to ward off the cognitive decline. Cognitive decline may not be inevitable.

Stress and Brain Longevity

Does stress cause mental decline? Mind-body research over the past 30 years has revealed a wealth of information about how our mind and body interact with one another. We used to think that the mind and brain were completely separate; however, we now know that they talk to one another constantly in the form of neuropeptides or protein chemicals that act as messengers between cells in the body.

Doctors' Orders

If you are easily annoyed, get angry or frustrated easily, feel powerless and hopeless, are self-critical and second-guess yourself, or frequently feel overwhelmed, you may be experiencing stress. Check with your doctor to find ways of reducing your stress response.

In the case of brain longevity, studies have shown that stress and depression may indeed contribute to decreased cognitive functioning. In *Brain Longevity* (Warner Books, 1997), Dr. Dharma Singh Khalsa reported on a Canadian study of elderly patients over a four-year period. The researchers found that patients with low stress (and therefore low cortisol levels) scored as well as their younger counterparts on memory tests, but patients who had increased stress and increased cortisol levels had a decline in memory and overall cognitive functioning. It is thought that high levels of cortisol are harmful to the brain and cause a decline in the neurons in the hippocampus, where the brain stores short-term memories. This may lead to cognitive decline.

Diseases Harmful to Brain Longevity

Certain factors inside the brain can lead to aging of the brain, but certain other diseases and conditions that can accelerate brain decline are treatable and reversible:

- Insomnia may lead to mental decline—especially chronic insomnia. Some evidence suggests that eight hours of regular sleep a night helps prevent memory loss.

- High blood pressure accelerates brain shrinkage and memory loss.

- Depression can cause changes in brain chemicals, causing some cognitive dysfunction. It can also cause a rise in cortisol levels that can lead to accelerated decline in the brain.

- Repetitive head trauma can lead to cognitive dysfunction later in life. This is often seen in boxers and others with traumatic brain injuries.

- Diabetes can lead to increased inflammation in the body, including the brain. Higher levels of blood sugars in the body are inflammatory—the change is not as pronounced with well-controlled diabetes. People with diabetes are found to have a higher incidence of Alzheimer's than the nondiabetic population.

- Atrial fibrillation, an abnormal heart rhythm, is a major cause of stroke and is often fatal.

Secrets of Successful Brain Longevity

Studies have shown that there are some lifestyle factors that are definitively associated with maintaining good brain functioning throughout the aging process. Physical activity, including aerobic exercise, seems to improve memory. So does mental exercise, such as new hobbies or new activities. Additionally, formal education is associated with less cognitive decline, perhaps due to continued learning creating strong neuron circuitry. A sense of control over one's life also seems to prevent cognitive decline.

Breathing Meditation

A cascade of chemical events occurs throughout the brain and the body during meditating that helps improve overall cognitive functioning. This includes a decrease in muscle tension and blood pressure, lowered cortisol levels, improved blood flow to the brain (as much as 25 percent), improved memory and alertness, and a strengthened immune system. Some evidence suggests that meditation slows down parts of the aging process.

The following breathing meditation is a good start for those who have never meditated, and it can be done sitting in a chair. Sit in your chair and bring up an image or memory of a peaceful space, such as a moonlit beach. Follow these steps:

1. Close your eyes and relax your posture.

2. Focus on your breathing only—let all other thoughts leave your mind.

3. Using your right hand, position yourself so that your thumb is over one nostril, and use your ring finger to alternately block off the other nostril.

4. Inhale slowly through the left nostril.

5. Exhale through the right nostril.

6. Inhale through the right nostril.

7. Breathe, alternating nostrils, blocking off one and then the other. Slow your pace until you develop a gentle rhythm, thinking only of the breathing. Continue for five minutes. Open your eyes.

Stroke

Strokes, or "brain attacks," occur when the brain is damaged by either the loss of blood supply to the brain from a clot or by bleeding into the brain tissue. Brain damage and death may result from either. Blood clots form in blood vessels that supply the brain. Bleeding into the brain occurs when a blood vessel bursts within the brain. In the United States, strokes are the leading cause of disability and the third leading cause of death. Each year, 700,000 people in the United States are victims of stroke, yet it is estimated that two thirds of all strokes could be prevented!

Doctors' Orders

Two million brain cells die every minute during a stroke. You can add years to your life by receiving prompt medical attention. Know the warning signs of stroke. Call 911 immediately if you experience a sudden onset of any of the following symptoms:

◆ Numbness or weakness of the face, arms, or legs—usually on one side of the body; facial weakness can show up as a tongue that deviates to the side, or a crooked smile

◆ Confusion

◆ Difficulty speaking or getting words out

◆ Trouble walking or sudden loss of balance

◆ Severe headache—"the worst headache of your life"

Alzheimer's Disease

Alzheimer's disease is the most common form of dementia and currently affects almost 5 million Americans. Alzheimer's disease is characterized by the deposition of protein plaque and tangled fibers in the brain. We don't yet know what causes Alzheimer's disease, though it is believed to have a genetic basis. However, environmental factors—your lifestyle—play an important role.

Prescription medications such as Namenda and Aricept may slow the progression of dementia once it is diagnosed, although benefits are not dramatic. Scientists are now trying to find medications that can prevent Alzheimer's disease, and research on alternative therapies is ongoing.

Risk Factors for Stroke and Dementia

Here are some risk factors for stroke and dementia. If you have any of the following, discuss prevention with your physician.

◆ *Increasing age:* Your risk for dementia increases with age.

◆ *Blockage of arteries, or atherosclerosis:* Increases the risk of strokes.

◆ *Smoking and alcohol use:* Smoking increases the risk of stroke. Too much alcohol increases the risk of dementia. Some studies show that moderate drinking—less than one drink a day for women and less than two drinks a day for men—may reduce the risk of dementia. However, if you do not drink, it is not recommended that you start.

◆ *High blood pressure:* Blood pressure that is persistently greater than 140/90 is a major risk factor for a stroke.

◆ *Atrial fibrillation:* An irregular heartbeat that is common in people over 75 years is another major risk factor for a stroke.

◆ *High cholesterol:* Increases your risk of strokes.

◆ *High homocysteine:* May be a risk for both Alzheimer's and strokes. Homocysteine is an amino acid produced in the body, usually as a by-product of consuming meat.

◆ *Diabetes:* Increases risks for both Alzheimer's and strokes.

◆ *Existing mild cognitive impairment:* Some pre-existing mild forgetfulness or memory decline increases the risk of developing dementia. The National Institute on Aging notes about 40 percent of those over 65 with mild cognitive impairment develop dementia within three years.

◆ *Physical inactivity:* Lack of exercise can increase your risk for stroke.

Some of the most important risk factors for stroke and dementia can be determined during a physical exam at your doctor's office. Working with your doctor, you can develop a strategy to lower your risk to average or even below average for your age.

Certain conditions can cause symptoms similar to dementia, and some of them are potentially reversible. These include …

◆ Medication reactions.

◆ Thyroid problems.

◆ Metabolic problems, such as low blood sodium or low blood sugar.

◆ Nutritional deficiencies, including vitamins B_1, B_6, and B_{12}, and folic acid.

◆ Dehydration.

◆ Infections.

◆ Subdural hematoma.

◆ Poisonings, including heavy metal poisoning.

◆ Brain tumors.

◆ Anoxia, or low blood supply states to the brain.

◆ Depression.

◆ Delirium.

Healthy Brain Practices

There is a great deal you can do to improve your brain's health. Eating a well-balanced, nutritious diet and exercising regularly are good ways to ensure optimal health and brain longevity.

Good Nutrition = Brain Food

A brain-healthy diet includes foods that have been shown to have nutrients that help the brain. It also avoids foods that promote high blood pressure, high cholesterol, and diabetes. And finally, it employs common sense and moderation.

The brain-healthy diet includes 5 to 10 servings of fruits and vegetables daily; fish or omega-3 fatty acids taken as a supplement; olive oil for cooking; black or green tea; whole grains; beans, other legumes, and nuts; and dark chocolate. The brain-healthy diet also limits or excludes red meat, excessive salt, trans fats, saturated or animal fats, high-glycemic foods, and overly processed foods. See Chapter 4 for more on good nutrition.

Longevity Facts

Know why you should eat certain foods. Eat apples and onions for their flavanoids; dark green leafy vegetables such as kale, spinach, and cooked tomatoes for their carotenes; and blueberries and pomegranates for their antioxidants.

Animal research studies suggest that curcumin, the pigment that gives the spice turmeric its yellow color, may slow the formation of Alzheimer's disease plaque in the brain. In mice brains, curcumin may even clear out pre-existing plaque. Some data also are starting to show that curcumin may play a role in the prevention of Alzheimer's. In India, turmeric is consumed by most people on a regular basis; it is also prescribed medicinally by Indian doctors. This might explain why India has one of the lowest rates of Alzheimer's disease in the world.

Curcumin is available in supplement pills. If you are at risk for Alzheimer's, consider taking curcumin in this form (check with your doctor). Several health experts recommend a dose of 500 mg to 1,000 mg per day. Finding ways to cook with turmeric is also a good way to consume curcumin. It can be added to many soups and vegetable dishes.

Exercise

Exercise your brain and your body, and do it regularly. Your brain will stay youthful and you will help prevent dementia. A 2003 *New England Journal of Medicine* study of 469 seniors found that participation in activities such as reading, playing board games, and playing musical instruments reduced the risk of dementia. Another 2006 study reported in the *Archives of Internal Medicine* showed that people who had a high level of physical function were three times less likely to get dementia, compared to those who fit the couch potato model.

Medications and Supplements That May Delay Dementia

Some herbs and supplements that show promise in prevention therapy for Alzheimer's include the following:

◆ Curcumin (mentioned earlier) works as an antioxidant and anti-inflammatory agent and may reduce plaque in the brain.

◆ Acetyl-L-carnitine (ALC) is an amino acid that helps to increase the amount of acetylcholine in your brain; the brains of Alzheimer's disease patients may be deficient in this.

◆ B vitamins, vitamins C and E, zinc, selenium, alpha-lipoic acid, and coenzyme-Q may help improve brain function.

◆ Fish oil contains omega-3s, which nourish your brain cells.

◆ Phosphatidylserine, the most abundant phospholipid in the brain, may be depleted in people with dementia. Some studies suggest that phosphatidylserine might improve cognition.

◆ Ginkgo is an herb that may improve blood flow in the brain.

◆ Arginine is an amino acid that can improve blood flow to the brain; it can also lower your blood pressure.

> **Doctors' Orders**
>
> Before you decide to include supplements in your diet, always check with your physician first. Some supplements may react with prescription medicines. Also, certain medical conditions may be aggravated by supplements, and there may be risk of serious reactions.

Additional Preventive Measures

Studies have shown that the following may be helpful in preventing dementia:

◆ *Lowering homocysteine levels:* High homocysteine has been shown to increase the risk of Alzheimer's almost three-fold and strokes by almost five-fold. B vitamins may help lower homocysteine levels. B vitamins can be easily obtained through a multivitamin.

◆ *Lowering cholesterol levels:* Cholesterol is involved in plaque formation in the brain. Statin medications may help prevent this.

◆ *Lowering blood pressure:* Certain studies have shown over 50 percent less dementia in people over 60 who were on medication treatment for their high blood pressure.

◆ *Controlling inflammation:* C reactive protein may help measure inflammation. A diet low in animal fats may help this.

◆ *Taking nonsteroidal anti-inflammatory drugs (NSAIDs):* In some studies, these medications reduced plaque formation and the incidence of both strokes and Alzheimer's disease. However, trials were stopped due to increased risk of heart attacks and hemorrhagic strokes in patients taking these medications.

Screening Tests

If you are having some memory problems and are not sure whether they're just related to normal stress or may be a sign of early dementia, it's time to go to the doctor for evaluation.

Many people are afraid of seeing the physician for memory loss, but *it's important to your brain longevity to get screened early.* If the cause of your cognitive decline is reversible, you can get it treated. If you are found to have evidence of a stroke, you will be able to proactively prevent subsequent strokes. If you do have Alzheimer's disease, medications are available to stabilize your condition for a period of time and ensure optimal brain outcomes. And research continues; important breakthroughs will be forthcoming!

When you are at the doctor's office, the following tests may be performed.

◆ *Patient history:* The doctor will ask questions regarding onset of symptoms and progression, and family members may be interviewed for further information.

◆ *Physical exam:* This will be done to check for other problems that may mimic dementia. The heart, lungs, and thyroid may be evaluated. A neurological exam may be done to check for signs of a stroke or movement disorders. Your reflexes and balance may be checked.

◆ *Mental status and neuropsychological exam:* A minimental status exam is used to check for cognitive dysfunction. A neuropsychological exam may help delineate types of cognitive decline and also separate them from stress, anxiety, and depression, which can also mimic dementia at times.

◆ *Lab work:* Labs may be drawn to check for reversible causes of dementia, including abnormalities in blood levels of sodium, glucose, thyroid hormone, and B_{12}. You may also be screened for tertiary syphilis.

◆ *Medication review:* Many medications, including pain medications, antidepressants, anxiety medications, sleep medications, or seizure medications, can alter cognitive functioning. A change in dose or medication interaction may sometimes be the source of increased confusion.

The "gold standard" for testing for dementia, especially Alzheimer's disease, is a brain biopsy at autopsy. This is obviously not a part of early screening for dementia, but other imaging studies can be done to check for causes of dementia and evaluate the state of the brain and blood vessels.

Carotid Ultrasound

A carotid ultrasound is a test that uses Doppler ultrasound to get a picture of the arteries leading to the brain. This is used to detect carotid stenosis, which is a narrowing of the carotid arteries. A carotid ultrasound may also pick up a dissection, which is a splitting between the layers of the artery wall.

A doctor may perform this test on you if you have risk factors for a stroke and a carotid "bruit" on a physical exam. This is an abnormal whooshing sound in your arteries that may be a sign of blockage. Some other risk factors that may lead to a carotid ultrasound are advanced age and the presence of other illnesses, such as high cholesterol, diabetes, or a family history of stroke or heart disease.

MRI/MRA

MRI stands for Magnetic Resonance Imaging, and this test uses a magnetic field to get pictures of soft tissues and bones inside the body. It is the most sensitive test to get a picture of the brain. An MRI is used to help diagnose brain tumors, aneurysms, strokes, signs of trauma, and other disorders of the nervous system, such as vasculitis and multiple sclerosis.

An MRA, or Magnetic Resonance Angiography, combines the MRI with contrast material to get a picture of the arteries. MRAs provide further information about the vessels leading to the brain (and those in the brain) and can reveal aneurysms, blockages, and dissections in the brain vessels.

New Research

Promising new therapies being studied for the treatment and prevention of Alzheimer's and other causes of dementia include the following:

- Vaccines to prevent the formation in the brain of plaque that leads to Alzheimer's

- Gene therapy and stem cell research to prevent degradation of brain neurons

- Vitamins to see if large doses of folic acid, B_{12}, and B_6 can prevent the rate of decline in Alzheimer's

- NSAID medications have proved promising in plaque reduction, but the increased risk of heart attack and hemorrhagic stroke has to be further evaluated

- Two medications, pentoxyfylline and propentofylline, may improve blood supply and reduce cell death in vascular dementia

Many supportive and preventive strategies exist for the treatment of dementia, but a cure has yet to been found. A study published in the November 18, 2002, issue of *The Archives of Neurology* found that the life span of people with Alzheimer's is dependent upon the age of the person when Alzheimer's is diagnosed. The study was performed by researchers at the Johns Hopkins Bloomberg School of Public Health. The results of this study indicate that the median survival of patients with Alzheimer's disease could range from nearly nine years for people diagnosed at age 65 to approximately three years for people diagnosed at age 90 years, according to Ronald Brookmeyer, Ph.D., professor of biostatistics at Johns Hopkins.

People diagnosed with Alzheimer's at age 65 could anticipate a 67 percent reduction in life span compared to those without Alzheimer's, while people diagnosed at age 90 could anticipate a 39 percent reduction in life span. There were no significant differences between men and women in survival after diagnosis of the disease.

The Least You Need to Know

- There is much you can do to prevent your risk of stroke; review your personal risk factors with your physician.

- Lifestyle interventions, such as a healthy diet, exercise, avoiding smoking, and keeping the brain active are key to pre-empting cognitive decline.

- Know the warning signs and symptoms of a stroke and seek immediate attention if they occur.

- See your doctor if you think you are starting to have memory loss. There are many potentially reversible conditions that may be causing your symptoms.

- Early diagnosis and treatment of all causes of dementia lead to the best outcomes. Being proactive in caring about your brain will improve its longevity.

Chapter 14

Say No to Diabetes

In This Chapter

- ◆ Understanding your risk for diabetes
- ◆ Your family history
- ◆ It's all about lifestyle
- ◆ Screenings and tests
- ◆ Diet—first line of defense
- ◆ Medical interventions

The Centers for Disease Control (CDC) reports that over 20 million Americans have adult-onset (type 2) diabetes and over 5 million of them are unaware of it. Diabetes is the sixth leading cause of death in the United States, and people with uncontrolled diabetes are also two to four times more likely to die of cardiovascular disease. In many cases, diabetes is the result of lifestyle choices. In this chapter, you'll learn strategies to help you avoid developing type 2 diabetes.

Understanding Diabetes

Diabetes is the common term for the medical condition known as *Diabetes mellitus,* in which the body's blood sugar is higher than normal. When we eat, our food is broken down in the intestines into glucose and other nutrients and absorbed into the bloodstream. From there, glucose is taken up by our tissues with the help of insulin, which is secreted from the pancreas. Glucose is the major source of fuel for much of the body. In diabetes, there is a problem with insulin production or utilization. Cells are unable to take up glucose; instead, levels increase in the blood. There are two main types of diabetes:

◆ *Type 1 diabetes:* This is an autoimmune disease in which the beta cells of the pancreas no longer make insulin because the body's immune system has destroyed them. This tends to occur in children but may also occur in adults.

◆ *Type 2 diabetes:* This is the most common form of diabetes and used to be known as adult-onset diabetes. This is highly linked to obesity and commonly occurs in adults; however, it is now being diagnosed in children. In type 2 diabetes, the body makes insulin but becomes resistant to it. This means that muscle, liver, and fat cells do not use insulin properly.

In this chapter, you'll learn about type 2 diabetes, which accounts for 90 to 95 percent of all diabetes cases. It's the kind you are the most likely to develop and the one you are most likely to be able to reverse.

Knowing Your Risk Factors

It is estimated that over 20 million people in the United States have type 2 diabetes. Of those, almost one third are undiagnosed. One study of over 80,000 nurses found that 9 out of 10 cases of type 2 diabetes among them was related to lifestyle. That's the bad news. The good news is that a research study completed in 2002, called the Diabetes Prevention Program, found that people 60 and older who followed a healthy lifestyle program greatly reduced their risk of developing diabetes by about 60 percent. If you find that you are at risk for diabetes, take appropriate action to increase your longevity.

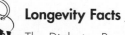

Longevity Facts

The Diabetes Prevention Program trial indicated that you can truly bypass the risk of getting diabetes, even if you are predisposed to it. Over the three years of the study, diet and exercise reduced the chances a person with mildly elevated blood sugars would develop diabetes. The diabetes medication metformin also reduced the risk, although less dramatically. What lifestyle measures were helpful in preventing diabetes? Eating less fat and fewer calories and exercising a total of 150 minutes a week. This group lost 7 percent of their body weight with these modifications. The take-home message? Small changes in diet and exercise, and modest changes in weight can have a huge impact in reducing your risk of developing a deadly disease.

Apple or Pear Shape?

The shape in which your body deposits fat has a lot to do with whether you are at risk of developing diabetes. People who have an apple-shaped body—weight distributed more around the middle and less on hips and thighs—tend to have an increased risk of developing diabetes. This is because abdominal obesity increases insulin resistance.

People who are pear-shaped, which is defined as a thinner waist and bigger hips and thighs, tend to have less of a tendency to develop diabetes, as compared to their apple-shaped counterparts. People with hourglass figures tend to fall into the pear-shaped category.

Unfortunately, you cannot change your body type from an apple to a pear, but you can decrease your waist size, if you're overweight. And because there is no proven method of spot reduction of fat, you'll have to do this the hard way—overall weight reduction will lead to a smaller waistline.

Syndrome X

Metabolic syndrome is also known as Syndrome X. It is a cluster of risk factors that, in combination, greatly increase the risk of diabetes and cardiovascular disease. The separate components of the syndrome include:

◆ Central obesity (an apple shape or a large waistline), where one's fat is localized around the middle—waist circumference of 40 inches or more in men, or 35 inches or more in women

◆ High blood pressure—130/85 or higher

- High triglycerides—above 150 mg per dl

- High-density lipoprotein (HDL) cholesterol—less than 40 mg per dl in men or less than 50 mg per dl in women

- Insulin resistance (the body can't properly control blood sugar levels)—fasting blood glucose (sugar) above 100 mg per dl

The diagnosis of metabolic syndrome or Syndrome X is made if an individual has three or more of these factors. If you have been diagnosed with Syndrome X, know that exercise, weight loss, and nutrition changes can reduce the risks associated with this condition and decrease the likelihood of developing type 2 diabetes, stroke, and heart disease. The exact cause of Syndrome X is unknown, but experts believe insulin resistance is the cause.

Family History and You

The tendency to develop type 2 diabetes can be inherited, although your risk depends to a greater extent on environmental factors, including your lifestyle, which we'll talk about in the next section. Knowing whether anyone in your family has a history of diabetes is important, because a family history of type 2 diabetes is one of the strongest risk factors for developing the disease. Interestingly enough, family history creates more of a tendency to diabetes in people living a Western lifestyle. In contrast, people who live in areas that have not become Westernized tend not to get type 2 diabetes, no matter how high their genetic risk.

Longevity Facts

Statistics show that if a parent has type 2 diabetes, the risk of the offspring getting diabetes is 1 in 7 if the parent was diagnosed before age 50 and 1 in 13 if the parent was diagnosed after age 50. If both parents have type 2 diabetes, risk in offspring is about 1 in 2.

Compared to the rest of the world, Americans and Europeans tend to eat more fat and refined carbohydrates, less fiber, and get too little exercise. Type 2 diabetes is more prevalent in people with these habits. Thus it can be said that type 2 diabetes tends to run in families—but this is in part due to learned poor lifestyle habits passed on to children.

Ethnicity also plays a role. Ethnic groups in the United States with the highest risk are African Americans, Mexican Americans, and Pima Indians and other Native Americans.

Minimizing Your Risk

Lifestyle is a big risk factor for diabetes, and making positive changes in lifestyle will greatly reduce your risk of developing this condition. Avoiding diabetes will definitely contribute to your longevity. If you find that you are at risk for diabetes, the following lifestyle changes can change your life! In addition to dietary recommendations covered later in the chapter, do the following:

◆ *Lose weight:* The great news is that even modest weight loss, in the range of 5 to 10 percent of body weight, can help restore your body's ability to use insulin and decrease insulin resistance.

◆ *Increase activity:* For example, a brisk 30-minute walk each day can result in weight loss, improved blood pressure, improved cholesterol levels, and a reduced risk of developing diabetes.

◆ *Limit alcohol intake:* Consume no more than one drink a day for women or two drinks for men. Alcohol has calories that can increase blood sugar and cause weight gain.

◆ *Stop smoking:* Smoking worsens the health consequences of the metabolic syndrome (Syndrome X). Many cessation plans are available, so talk to your doctor about ways to quit smoking. (See Chapter 12 for more information.)

Knowing Your Diabetes Numbers

Knowing your diabetes numbers and being able to determine your chances of developing diabetes can help you make important lifestyle changes that will enhance longevity. People generally start showing a tendency toward elevated blood sugars years before they are formally diagnosed with diabetes. If you are on top of your numbers, you will know if you have pre-diabetes, or elevated blood sugars that are above normal but not high enough to be classified as diabetes.

If you are diagnosed with pre-diabetes, there is much you can do to perhaps delay or even prevent developing diabetes. Three blood tests are available to diagnose diabetes: a fasting plasma glucose test, an oral glucose tolerance test, and a random plasma glucose test. An elevated reading on any of these can lead to a diagnosis of diabetes.

Fasting Plasma Glucose Test

This test is done after fasting, which is defined as not eating anything for at least eight hours. This test is generally done in the morning after not having had anything to eat after dinner the previous night. Water or black coffee or tea without cream or sugar prior to the test is permitted. Any beverages with cream or sugar will falsely elevate the numbers.

A normal reading on the Fasting Plasma Glucose Test is 99 and below; pre-diabetes (also known as impaired fasting glucose) ranges between 100 to 125, and diabetes is diagnosed at 126 and above.

Oral Glucose Tolerance Test

This test may be more sensitive for diagnosing pre-diabetes, but it takes longer to administer and is more of a hassle for patients. It requires a fast for at least eight hours before the test. The plasma glucose is then measured immediately before and two hours after you drink a liquid containing 75 g of glucose.

A score of 139 and below is considered normal, pre-diabetes scores fall between 140 and 199, and diabetes is diagnosed with a score of 200 or above. The diagnosis is confirmed by repeating the test on a different day.

This test is rarely used these days, as it is inconvenient to perform. The exception is testing for gestational diabetes.

Random Plasma Glucose Test

This test can be run from blood drawn at a lab or from a finger prick test at the doctor's office. Diabetes is diagnosed with a level of over 200, especially in the presence of symptoms of increased urination, thirst, or unexplained weight loss.

Assess Your Risk

If you answer yes to any of the following statements, you may want to discuss diabetes testing with your doctor:

◆ I am 45 years old or older.

◆ I am overweight or obese.

◆ I have a family history of diabetes (parent, brother, or sister).

♦ I am from a race that has an increased prevalence of diabetes (African American, American Indian, Asian American, Pacific Islander, Hispanic American, or Latino).

♦ I am female and either had gestational diabetes or gave birth to a baby weighing more than 9 pounds.

♦ My blood pressure is high (over 140/90).

♦ My cholesterol levels are above normal.

♦ I am inactive (exercise less than three times a week).

♦ I have an apple-shaped body.

> **Doctors' Orders**
>
> Warning signs of type 2 diabetes include frequent urination; extreme hunger or thirst; fatigue and irritability; frequent infections, including skin, bladder, or vaginal infections; and numbness or tingling in your feet or hands. Even with no symptoms you may still be at risk.

Recommended Screenings

Very few diabetics actually die of diabetes; rather, mortality is associated with complications of untreated or poorly controlled diabetes. If you are a diabetic and want to increase your longevity, make sure you continue to monitor your condition to prevent diabetes-related complications. If you have diabetes, be sure to keep current on the necessary screenings, as advised by your doctor.

Heart Screenings

Two of every three diabetes patients die of heart disease or stroke. If you have diabetes, you can maximize your longevity by maintaining good cardiovascular health. This includes watching your weight, blood pressure, cholesterol, and having regular checkups—so that early high blood pressure can be controlled before you suffer a stroke. This also means not smoking!

Diabetics are more likely to have sudden heart attacks. Therefore, if you experience any change in your health, see your doctor to rule out heart disease. Symptoms could include increasing weakness, dizziness, exercise intolerance, palpitations, nausea, back, shoulder, neck, or jaw pain. (See Chapters 10 and 13 for more on heart disease and stroke, respectively.)

Regular Skin Care

One-third of all diabetics have skin-related problems, many of which can be prevented if treated early. If left untreated, skin infections and wounds can lead to more serious complications, including cellulitis or amputations. Keep your skin clean and dry. Treat cuts immediately and consult a dermatologist if your skin problems do not resolve.

Foot Screenings

Keep your feet healthy. Check your feet every day and have a foot exam at least once a year from your doctor. You can also choose to see a podiatrist, especially if you have corns, calluses, or cracked heels. If you have toenails that are thickened and hard to trim, a podiatrist will help you with that. Always wear shoes to avoid unintended foot injuries that may lead to infections. By avoiding ill-fitting shoes, you will avoid blisters that may worsen to infections. Finally, wash and dry your feet every day; if you have athlete's foot, get this treated. Treat all infections early—don't wait for them to spread.

Eye Screenings

Diabetics have four times the risk of retinopathy as those who have normal blood glucose. Retinopathy is an abnormal growth of blood vessels in the eyes that happens in response to elevated glucose and can lead to low vision or blindness. If you have retinopathy and want to improve your vision longevity, see a doctor regularly and keep your sugars under tight control—you will reduce your progression of retinopathy by 50 percent!

Diabetics should see an ophthalmologist or optometrist yearly for a dilated eye exam—especially all diabetics age 30 or older.

Oral Screening

Diabetes can make plaque and gingivitis worse, as it impairs the body's ability to fight infections. It can also worsen oral infections and make it harder for the body to heal after oral surgery. Poor oral health may also aggravate inflammation and cardiovascular disease. Keeping on top of your dental care is key to avoiding worsening oral hygiene. This includes brushing regularly, flossing regularly, and seeing the dentist regularly.

Dietary Considerations

There is much fascinating research on the impact of various foods on diabetes. By incorporating a balanced diet into your treatment plan, your diabetes will be better controlled. Death and complications from diabetes drastically decrease when diabetes is well controlled. So how do you eat your way to a long life if you are a diabetic? Eat food in its least processed, most natural form, with a diet low in processed sugars, refined carbohydrates, and animal fats. There is a great deal you can do in the food department to decrease your chances of developing type 2 diabetes and increasing your longevity.

> ### Words to the Wise
>
> *Diabetes Care,* a journal published by the American Diabetes Association, reported on a study that compared a standard American Diabetes Association diet to a low-fat, low-sugar vegan diet. A vegan diet does not contain animal or dairy products. The study found that people on the vegan diet lost more weight and controlled their diabetes better than those on the standard diabetic diet. Why? It's easier to control the caloric content and portion size of our meals when we eat more fruits and vegetables—hence the success of the vegan diet. Consider going vegan if you're a diabetic!

Minimize Sucrose

Sucrose (sugar) causes higher triglycerides, higher blood glucose, and harmful cholesterol levels. A 2002 study suggested that a high level of sugar consumption may also reduce levels of HDL cholesterol, the "good" cholesterol.

Consider Cinnamon

Several studies suggest that ¼ to ½ teaspoon of cassia cinnamon a day can lower blood sugar and cholesterol levels by up to 30 percent. The data on the efficacy of cinnamon, however, is mixed. Cassia cinnamon, also known as Chinese cinnamon or *Cinnamomum aromatica*, is the same cinnamon found in the spice department of your local grocery store.

> ### Doctors' Orders
>
> Talk to your doctor before beginning to take cinnamon if you have adult-onset diabetes or high cholesterol. This is important especially if you are on medications, as you may need an adjustment in your medication dosages.

Cinnamon acts like an insulin sensitizer, making insulin work more effectively. This is similar to how some prescription medications currently used for adult-onset diabetes work. Cinnamon is only effective for adult onset (type 2 diabetes). It does not work for juvenile (type 1) diabetes.

When adding cinnamon to your diet, you may want to pass on the cinnamon rolls and apple pie—foods high in fat and sugar content. Instead, add cinnamon to your oatmeal, coffee, or tea.

Take Fiber

Soluble fiber supplements, such as those that contain psyllium, may be beneficial. Psyllium is taken from the husk of a seed grown in India and can be found in laxatives and breakfast cereals. A 2002 study demonstrated that patients with type 2 diabetes who consumed psyllium (Plantaben) for breakfast for 11 weeks experienced lower total and "bad cholesterol," or LDL cholesterol levels. There was no difference in glucose levels. Psyllium may increase gas and bloating, however.

Chromium

Chromium has been shown to improve blood sugar control in some diabetics, but the studies on this supplement are not that strong in favor of its effectiveness. It appears at this stage that chromium may help decrease blood sugars in people who have a chromium deficiency. For those who don't, however, it may not do much of anything. Thus, at this stage, the American Diabetes Association recommends chromium only for patients with documented chromium deficiency. Talk to your doctor about this supplement before taking it.

Fat Awareness

There is a growing focus of research on foods that cause inflammation and thus worsen diseases such as diabetes. It has been found that there is possible harm from end-products of the chemical reaction between sugar and protein—called advanced glycation end-products (AGEs). This reaction happens when animal fats are cooked at high temperatures. On the other hand, low, slow cooking produces fewer AGEs. Steaming or cooking food in water does not produce these chemicals.

Tank the trans fats. Trans fatty acids are manufactured fats created during a process called hydrogenation, which is aimed at stabilizing polyunsaturated oils to prevent them from becoming rancid. Trans fats are solid at room temperature and keep packaged foods—such as cookies and crackers—crispy. They are used in cooking and frying of fast foods. Trans fats are particularly dangerous for the heart and may even pose a risk for certain cancers (see Chapter 11). Studies report that high consumption of these fats reduces HDL and raises LDL cholesterol levels, has harmful effects on the linings of the arteries, and may increase the risk for type 2 diabetes.

Words to the Wise
Above all, it's important to stay committed to eating well. One study of people with type 2 diabetes compared diabetics who followed a high-carbohydrate/high-fiber diet, a low-fat diet, and a weight management diet. After 18 months all groups showed better cholesterol and diabetes numbers. It was concluded that the positive benefits of the diets were derived not from the specific regimens, but because the people in the study were focused and stuck with them. Thus, healthy nutrition works when you are committed to it.

White Meat, Not Red

A large 2006 study found that red meat increases the risk of women developing type 2 diabetes. This is thought to be due to high iron levels in red meat. Another 2006 study suggested that replacing red meat with white meat improves kidney function and cholesterol levels in patients with diabetic kidney problems.

No to Vitamin E

A 2005 *Journal of the American Medical Association* study found that diabetics who take vitamin E supplements actually had an increased risk of heart failure.

Yes to Java

Good news for the coffee addicts out there! Multiple studies have noted an association between coffee consumption and reduced risk for developing type 2 diabetes. A 2006 study of 29,000 post-menopausal women showed a positive effect of caffeine in reducing diabetes. In this study, women who drank at least six cups of coffee a day (either regular or decaf) were 22 percent less likely to develop type 2 diabetes as compared to noncoffee drinkers. (Of course, you want to drink coffee in moderation; six cups of coffee a day would have most people climbing the walls!)

Another study on decaffeinated coffee showed that women who drank at least six cups a day of decaf were 33 percent less likely to develop diabetes than women who did not drink coffee. The mechanism of the coffee on improving diabetes is unknown, but may be due to an antioxidant effect. Similar effects on improvement in diabetes have been shown with oolong tea (a particular type of fermented tea).

Medications

Initial medication treatment of type 2 diabetes usually consists of prescription oral medication. These can be of the following types:

- *Sulfonylureas:* Stimulate the pancreas to make more insulin.

- *Biguanides:* Decrease the amount of glucose produced by the liver.

- *Thiazolidinediones:* Increase the body's sensitivity to insulin.

- *Alpha-glucosidase inhibitors:* Slow the absorption of starches.

- *Meglitinides:* Stimulate the pancreas to produce more insulin.

- *DPP4 medications:* Stimulate the pancreas to make insulin only when food is eaten.

As type 2 diabetes progresses, these medications may become ineffective, and blood sugar levels may start being uncontrolled, even with medication treatment. Your physician may discuss transitioning to insulin at that time.

Doctors' Orders _____

Low blood sugar reactions can be life-threatening. These can happen in diabetics for various reasons, including not eating enough or soon enough, overexertion, overmedicating, and alcohol ingestion. Symptoms can include shakiness, dizziness, sweating, lightheadedness, palpitations, confusion, and anxiety. If you experience these symptoms, check your blood sugar; if it is less than 70, take 15 g of carbs, which can include ½ cup of juice, 1 cup of milk, 1 to 2 teaspoons of sugar, hard candy, or glucose tablets.

There are certain prescription medications, such as gabapentin and tricyclic antidepressants, that help block the sensation of pain at the nerve ending, or neuropathy. Peripheral neuropathy can be caused by longstanding uncontrolled diabetes but may also be caused by chronic alcoholism, nutritional deficiencies, or certain infections. Various alternative treatments have been used for neuropathy, including megavitamins, magnets, acupuncture, and chiropractic manipulation.

There is not an abundance of data on the effectiveness of alternative treatments for peripheral neuropathy, although patients who use these measures report a reduction of pain about 25 percent of the time. Certain vitamins, such as thiamine, B_6, and B_{12}, have been found beneficial when a deficiency of these vitamins exists. Giving alpha-lipoic acid orally or intravenously 600 mg to 1,200 mg per day seems to reduce symptoms of peripheral neuropathy in diabetes patients. Treating the underlying cause if one is found (controlling diabetes or stopping drinking alcoholic beverages) will be beneficial.

The Least You Need to Know

- One third of those with diabetes do not know they have it.

- Type 2 diabetes can be anticipated by knowing your personal risk factors.

- Many risk factors for diabetes, including obesity, can be reversed by lifestyle measures such as regular exercise.

- Decreasing your intake of saturated fats, processed foods, and refined carbohydrates will help prevent diabetes.

- For those with diabetes, good heart health and stroke prevention can reduce mortality by two thirds.

Chapter 15

Musculoskeletal Health

In This Chapter

- ◆ Bone strength and long life
- ◆ Another reason to exercise
- ◆ The spoilers
- ◆ Risk factors for osteoporosis
- ◆ Osteoporosis or osteoarthritis?
- ◆ Arthritis: the nation's leading cause of disability

The musculoskeletal system refers to your muscles and your skeleton, of course. In this chapter, you'll learn all you need to know about keeping your bones and joints in good working condition and operating at optimal strength over the course of your life span. You want to avoid joint wear and tear and fractures. You also want to lead a pain-free life and have enough strength to enjoy normal daily activities and hobbies. Optimizing your musculoskeletal health is the starting point to accomplishing this.

Keeping Your Bones Strong

The musculoskeletal system is the structural foundation for the rest of the body, and strong bones are the foundation of this system. Keeping your musculoskeletal system strong helps keep away common diseases and injuries, such as osteoporosis, arthritis, and fractures. No matter what your age, it's never too late to optimize your bone health, and there are proven benefits from keeping your bones and joints strong and healthy.

You can think about bone health from two perspectives. The first is bone density, which determines the thickness and strength of the bones. Inadequate bone strength is referred to as osteopenia or osteoporosis. The second is pain and debilitation in the joints. This is often diagnosed as arthritis. The Centers for Disease Control (CDC) reports that one in five adults and 50 percent of adults age 65 and older have received a diagnosis of arthritis, which can include rheumatoid arthritis, gout, and lupus. With arthritis affecting such a significant percentage of the population, it has merited serious attention from researchers and physicians. While research continues, doctors do know that certain lifestyle changes and dietary supplements can help.

Calcium

Your body needs adequate calcium if it's going to function optimally. Adolescence and young adulthood is a critical time for taking in sufficient quantities of calcium in order to establish optimal bone density by age 30, when bone density begins to decline.

What does this translate to for the average person? Adults under 50 need 1,000 mg of calcium daily, and those over 50 need 1,200 to 1,500 mg of calcium daily. Generally, two 500 mg calcium supplements that contain vitamin D, taken with food, is a good way to incorporate calcium into your daily regimen. If you want to incorporate calcium into your diet naturally, good sources of calcium in food include:

- Dairy, such as low-fat or nonfat milk, cheese (including goat cheese), and yogurt

- Dark-green vegetables, including bok choi and broccoli

- Calcium-fortified foods, such as orange juice, cereal, oatmeal, bread, soy beverages, tofu products, and nuts (including almonds)

- Canned fish with bones, such as salmon or sardines

Vitamin D

Vitamin D is increasingly recognized as a key player in maintaining bone strength, and some studies are beginning to suggest that some of us may be deficient in vitamin D. The recommended daily allowance (RDA) of vitamin D is 400 to 800 International Units (IU) for those under 50, and 800 to 1,200 IU for those over 50. Vitamin D_3, cholecalciferol, is the best form of vitamin D to help the bones; it's found in foods such as fortified milk, saltwater fish, egg yolks, and supplements.

> **Doctors' Orders**
>
> Foods that have been supplemented with vitamin D don't always contain the amounts the label says. Taking supplemental vitamin D is one way to ensure you receive the recommended daily allowance.

Sunlight is a good, natural source of vitamin D. Vitamin D is manufactured in your skin when it's exposed to the sun. The body's ability to do this declines as you age if you live in more northern latitudes, and also during nonsummer months. Unfortunately, most of us spend our days inside, and when we do venture out, we slather on the sunscreen, which inhibits our body's ability to make vitamin D. However, keep in mind that sunlight exposure increases your risk of skin cancer. See Chapter 17 for more discussion on this.

So what should you do if you are concerned about your vitamin D status? Consider getting your blood level checked. An ideal level is probably *at least* 50 nanomoles per liter. Taking 1,000 units a day total of vitamin D (from food and supplements together) should be enough to achieve this. The maximum recommended intake is 2,000 units a day.

Other vitamins and supplements (see Chapter 7 for more information) that may be important or useful for bone health include:

- Vitamin K
- Potassium
- Magnesium
- Manganese
- Copper
- Ipriflavone
- Soy

- DHEA

- Zinc

Intriguing supplements and foods being researched for their benefits for bone health are boron, tea, and coffee!

Exercise for Your Bones

Weight-bearing exercise is key here. This helps form strong bones—no matter what age you start. Good exercises for bone strengthening include walking, dancing, jogging, jumping rope, weight lifting, soccer, basketball, and racquet sports. And when in doubt: walk, walk, walk!

Only 16 percent of people who are either underweight or of normal weight are diagnosed with arthritis. This number jumps with weight gain. Approximately 66 percent of adults with arthritis are overweight or obese. Engaging in moderate exercise three times a week, however, can reduce the risk of arthritis-related disability in older adults with knee osteoarthritis by 47 percent.

Longevity Facts

The fundamental secret for joint longevity? Lose that excess weight! Studies have shown that weight loss of as little as 11 pounds reduces the risk of developing knee osteoarthritis among women by 50 percent.

You should also do stability exercises to decrease the potential for falls and fractures. These include exercise regimens such as Pilates for core body strengthening and tai chi for gait stability. Pool exercises are great for those who can't do regular exercises without pain. A heated pool works wonders on those aching joints. However, while swimming has many health benefits, it is not a weight-bearing exercise and will not work to increase bone density.

Breaking Bad Bone Habits

Smoking and excessive alcohol consumption have been found to decrease bone density. Excessive dieting, poor dietary intake of calcium, and anorexia can also increase your risk of thinning bones. Eat a well-balanced diet; get your calcium; and if you smoke, make that effort to quit (see Chapter 12).

Smoking and Bone Health

Smoking has many detrimental effects on musculoskeletal health and will decrease the longevity of your joints. Fractures in smokers take longer to heal because of the harmful effects of nicotine on the production of bone-forming cells. Smoking impairs lung function—and there is less oxygen available for muscles used in physical activity and exercise. Thus, smokers have three times the amount of shortness of breath than nonsmokers and find that they cannot run or walk as fast or as far as their nonsmoking counterparts. Research has shown that smoking also affects the musculoskeletal system in the following ways:

◆ Smoking increases the risk of developing osteoporosis. (See the section on osteoporosis later in this chapter.)

◆ Smoking increases the risk of a hip fracture. Elderly smokers have a 41 percent increase in the rate of hip fractures.

◆ Smoking leads to an increased incidence of traumatic injuries (such as sprains or fractures) as compared to nonsmokers.

◆ Smokers have a higher postsurgical rate of complications than nonsmokers.

Unanticipated Side Effects

Acid-blocking medications—specifically, proton pump inhibitors such as Prilosec—may be linked to bone fractures. According to a recent study published in the *Journal of the American Medical Association*, people who took proton pump inhibitors for over a year had a 44 percent higher risk of hip fractures. Higher doses of these medications were associated with higher rates of fractures.

Proton pump inhibitors should not replace lifestyle changes to decrease acid reflux. Eating balanced meals; losing excess weight; decreasing stress; avoiding eating within three hours before sleeping; avoiding tight belts; and avoiding acidic foods such as citrus, tomatoes, and alcohol can all decrease acid reflux. If despite making these changes you continue to have significant *GERD*, then appropriate use of acid-blocking medication may still be an appropriate option for you.

def•i•ni•tion

GERD is the acronym for gastro-esophageal reflux disease, also known as chronic heartburn. Signs of GERD may include epigastric pain, metallic taste in the mouth, and burning in the esophagus.

Soft Drinks/Soft Bones

Consuming soft drinks has been linked to decreased bone mineral density (BMD), which is a number that tells how dense your bones are. Unfortunately, it appears that it does not matter if the cola is diet, regular, or noncarbonated—all decrease BMD.

A recent study in the *American Journal of Clinical Nutrition* studied the effects of soda drinking on over 2,000 men and women. The study found that people who drank less than one cola a month had greater bone density than those who drank daily cola. What is interesting is people who drank more cola did not drink less milk, so a decreased milk intake is not the reason that cola drinkers have thinner bones. It is thought the reason behind the decreased BMD in cola drinkers is two-fold: caffeine in cola may be linked to osteoporosis, and cola contains phosphoric acid, which decreases the calcium in the body by impairing its absorption and increasing its excretion.

If you are at risk for osteoporosis, you should consider decreasing your intake of sodas. Choose water first.

Thinning Bones: Osteoporosis

In 2000, 10 percent of adults in the United States aged 50 years or older had osteoporosis. Whereas we may think of this as a women's disease, osteoporosis affects more than 2 million men in the United States.

Still, women are more likely than men to develop osteoporosis. Women have a smaller stature than men, with smaller, thinner bones. After menopause, bone loss in women greatly exceeds that in men. Women lose bone mass rapidly in the first 6 to 12 months after menopause, due to the precipitous decline in production of the hormone estrogen, which normally supports the bones. After this initial period, the decline slows. By age 65, women and men tend to lose bone mass at the same rate. Part of this is due to the declining production of the hormone testosterone in both men and women as they age. This can lead to increased bone loss and a greater risk of developing osteoporosis.

Are you at risk for osteoporosis? You may be and not be aware of it. The National Osteoporosis Foundation (www.NOF.org) provides a self-survey to help you determine your risk factors. Being aware of your risk factors can help you take preventive action.

◆ Do you have a small, thin frame and/or are you Caucasian or Asian?

◆ Have you or a member of your immediate family broken a bone as an adult?

- Are you a post-menopausal woman?

- Have you had an early or surgically induced menopause?

- Have you taken high doses of thyroid medication or used glucocorticoids (prednisone, for example) for more than three months?

- Have you taken, or are you taking, immunosuppressive medications or chemotherapy to treat cancer?

- Is your diet low in dairy products or other sources of calcium?

- Do you smoke cigarettes or drink alcohol to excess?

The more times you answer yes, the greater your risk for developing osteoporosis. In addition, medications such as chronic oral steroids or anticonvulsants can increase your risk of osteoporosis. A height loss of 1 inch or 2 inches may also be an indicator for osteoporosis, as can kyphosis, or the "buffalo hump" on the base of the back of the neck. See your doctor for more information.

Screening for Bone Mineral Density (BMD)

How can you tell if you have thinning bones? Contrary to popular belief, thinning bones do not cause bone pain, unless you get a fracture. Osteoporosis is a silent disease, and the only way to check for it is through a DEXA, or a bone density scan.

The major organizations that make recommendations for health screening in the United States do not recommend *routine* screening for osteoporosis in adults until age 60 to 65. If someone has significant risk factors for osteoporosis, such as chronic steroid or seizure medicine use, then screening is done at an earlier age. This is because most of the data we have regarding osteoporosis treatment has been done in older women; data regarding any benefit in younger women is sparse.

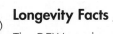 **Longevity Facts**

The DEXA evaluates your bone strength. This is a simple x-ray test that measures the thickness of the bones and can calculate if your bones are thinning. A DEXA can also help determine risk of fracture and rate of bone loss. Medicare pays for a bone density exam every two years.

Once you have been diagnosed with osteoporosis, your doctor may advise you to take a certain class of medications called bisphosphonates. These medications reduce the rate of bone loss and have been shown to reduce the risk of fractures. Even if you are on a bisphosphonate to treat your thinning bones, you still need to maintain an adequate intake of calcium and vitamin D and keep up your weight-bearing exercises. For osteoporosis *prevention*, hormones such as estrogen and parathyroid hormone may be prescribed.

Preventing Falls and Improving Your Longevity

Among Americans age 65 and older, fall-related injuries are the leading cause of accidental death. The CDC and National Osteoporosis Foundation (NOF) report that people who have a hip fracture are 5 to 20 percent more likely to die than their counterparts over the first year following injury. They also are 15 to 25 percent more likely to be in long-term care institutions a year after their injury. Osteoporosis is related to the vast majority of hip fractures. Other factors that lead to falls as people get older are slowed reflexes, decreased balance and stability, and weakened musculoskeletal strength.

To lessen your risk of falls, do muscle-strengthening exercises, get your vision checked regularly, and practice balance exercises daily. You also want to watch out for medications that may increase your risk of falls, including tranquilizers, sleeping medications, and some blood pressure medications. Finally, keep your environment safe to prevent the risk of falls. This includes keeping your house free of clutter, keeping it well lighted, and avoiding throw rugs. (See Chapter 2 for more on what you can do to prevent falls.)

Bisphosphonates and Osteonecrosis

Recent data has suggested that the class of drugs commonly used to treat osteoporosis, the bisphosphonates, can cause osteonecrosis or deterioration of the jaw bones. This is usually only seen in the intravenous forms of these drugs, which are generally reserved for patients with cancer in the bones. Oral forms of these drugs, which include Fosamax, Actonel, and Boniva, have rarely been associated with this disorder. However, given the possibility of this, it is now recommended that you see your dentist to complete any necessary dental work involving extractions or implants before you start these drugs.

Osteoporosis vs. Osteoarthritis

It's easy to confuse these two terms. Osteoporosis refers to *thinning* of the bones. Osteoarthritis, on the other hand, refers to the *wear and tear* of the joints. This is similar to the brake pads wearing down on your car. Both osteoarthritis and osteoporosis have to do with the musculoskeletal system, and both happen as we get older, but the similarity stops there. Thinning bones are caused, in large part, by poor nutrition and poor health.

Arthritis

Arthritis has a lot to do with repetitive damage to the joints. Let's explore secrets to avoiding wear and tear in your joints—preventing osteoarthritis.

Arthritis means more than gnarled knuckles and swollen joints. It's painful and can take the joy out of living. If you can no longer pursue the activities that have given you pleasure, life becomes difficult. Losing joint function can turn into a serious, chronic disability. While certain medications can help, avoiding arthritis, if at all possible, is infinitely preferable.

def•i•ni•tion

Arthritis refers to inflammation of the joints and is a grab-bag term that includes over 100 different types of conditions. These include gout, osteoarthritis, and autoimmune arthritis such as rheumatoid arthritis. Osteoarthritis is one of the most common types of painful joint conditions.

According to the CDC, arthritis is the nation's leading cause of disability, and it is not just an "old person's" disease—almost two thirds of people with arthritis are younger than 65. Almost 50 million Americans suffer from arthritis, and this condition is a source of disability for 19 million of them. That translates roughly into one in five Americans. Arming yourself with the knowledge on prevention and treatment of arthritis will add years to your joint life.

Secrets of Preventing Arthritis

At any point in your life, it's possible to make positive changes to limit the effects arthritis might have on your health span. The CDC recommends early diagnosis and appropriate management of arthritis to decrease pain and improve function. There are many ways you can help yourself and your joints!

Continue to be active. Keeping the core body in good condition decreases stress on the joints. Some people falsely believe they should stop exercising if their joints hurt. Actually, becoming sedentary makes things worse. However, it is wise to do exercises that are low impact and that do not worsen the joint pain. This may mean walking on a treadmill as opposed to running on hard pavement. Also, swimming, cycling, and pool therapy are easier on the joints than high-impact activities.

Protect your joints. This includes avoiding repetitive trauma (e.g., running on hard pavement). And make sure you wear good footwear. High heels are bad for the joints, but did you know chunky heels are bad, too? Flat heels with good arch support are best.

Watch your weight and know your Body Mass Index (BMI). Just 10 to 15 extra pounds put you at higher risk of osteoarthritis of the knees, hips, and spine. One pound of extra weight is equal to 2 to 3 extra pounds of stress on the knees.

If you begin having joint pain, see your doctor for an accurate diagnosis and an appropriate treatment regimen. The doctor may perform a symptom-directed history and physical exam. Tests for joint pain may include labs such as Sedimentation Rate, Rheumatoid Factor, and antinuclear antibody (ANA) to check for autoimmune disease. An x-ray of the affected joint may also be done for evaluating arthritis. Other tests that may be done include joint aspiration (arthrocentesis), MRI, CT scan, or a bone scan.

If you need medication, start out with acetaminophen (Tylenol) as an analgesic. For more severe pain, your doctor may advise anti-inflammatories, including ibuprofen and naproxen. If you experience stomach upset with these medications, COX 2 inhibitors, such as Celebrex, may be an option, as they provide the anti-inflammatory effect without some of the stomach side effects.

Discuss all medications and supplements with your doctor prior to starting them.

Other treatments that may have some benefit in helping decrease the pain of osteoarthritis include:

- Topical rubs, including arnica, camphor, and capsaicin

- Oral supplements, including glucosamine, chondroitin, SAMe, MSM, gelatin, and essential fatty acids

- Herbs, including boswellia, cat's claw, devil's claw, ginger, myrrh, turmeric, and white willow bark

Exercising with Arthritis

Exercising with arthritis is like the proverbial catch-22. You are not exercising due to knee pain, and the lack of exercise is contributing to your obesity, which worsens your arthritic pain. So how do you break out of this cycle? Here are some tips:

◆ Start slowly but start moving. Start with range-of-motion exercises that do not put any strain on your knees.

◆ Engage a personal trainer or physical therapist to assist you in exercises that stabilize your knees and strengthen your quadriceps and hamstrings.

◆ Focus on activities that minimize microtrauma (e.g., walk or use the exercise bike instead of running, or utilize the treadmill instead of walking on hard pavement).

◆ Exercise in two 15-minute blocks during the day instead of one 30-minute block.

◆ Utilize the pool for fat burning—if you can't swim well, do aerobic exercises in the shallow end of the pool.

◆ You can try Pilates for core body strengthening, tai chi for stability, or yoga for enhancing flexibility.

◆ Avoid activities that cause increased knee pain or joint swelling.

◆ Apply heat to painful joints prior to activity and ice after to reduce the swelling.

Physical therapy, occupational therapy with the use of a TENS unit, or an ultrasound can all be beneficial in helping the inflammation of arthritis.

If you want to lose weight, combine a regular exercise program based on the previous recommendations with a healthy diet. Go to www.mypyramid.gov for free personalized caloric intake recommendations based on your age and level of physical activity.

Dietary Recommendations

You want to create a diet that incorporates foods that are anti-inflammatory for the joints. To do this, put an emphasis on eating more fruits and vegetables, at least 5 to 10 servings a day.

Include fish in your diet. Choose cold water fish, such as salmon, which is rich in omega-3 oils. Or you can add flax seed oil—another source of omega-3 to your diet—at around a teaspoon per day. Omega-3 oils are anti-inflammatory oils and help to reduce pain.

Foods that should be minimized are highly processed foods, especially highly processed snack foods or prepackaged foods rich in trans fats or hydrogenated oils.

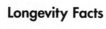

Longevity Facts _____

The USDA ranks the following foods as antioxidants, and these foods may be helpful in reducing inflammation in painful joints: blueberries, kale, strawberries, spinach, Brussels sprouts, plums, broccoli, beets, and red grapes. The following foods may cause inflammation, and *avoiding* these foods may help reduce joint pain: corn, dairy, wheat, citrus, dairy, tomatoes, yeast, and soybeans. The data on these is inconclusive, however, and should be personally evaluated.

The bottom line is that eating foods in their nonprocessed natural states and avoiding red meats and saturated fats is key to reducing joint pain. (See Chapter 4 for more on nutrition.)

When All Else Fails

If you have arthritis and you have tried to get to your ideal weight, strengthened your muscles, tried anti-inflammatory medications, and your joints are still sore, you and your doctor still have options.

Steroid injections into the joint space reduce the inflammation in the joint. However, steroids can cause further cartilage and joint deterioration, so excessive steroid injections are not recommended.

Hyaluronic acid injections, including Synvisc, Hyalgan, Supartz, and Orthovisc, function much like a lubricant for the knees and are usually given in a series of three to five injections.

Narcotic analgesics such as codeine can help with pain control, and muscle relaxers may help with the associated muscular pain that may occur with arthritis.

Surgical options include arthroscopic surgery and joint replacement. Joints such as the shoulders and the knees may be amenable to noninvasive surgery that may help to clean up some of the cartilage irregularities and thus decrease pain. When all else fails, it may be time for a brand-new joint. You don't want to rush to this step, because artificial joints have a limited life span and the earlier you get them, the greater the likelihood you will need a replacement joint.

The Least You Need to Know

- ◆ To keep your bones strong at any age, get enough calcium and vitamin D and exercise regularly.

- ◆ Smoking, routine use of acid-blocking medications, and excessive consumption of alcohol and soft drinks decrease bone density.

- ◆ Osteoporosis refers to thinning bones, which can increase your chances of a fracture.

- ◆ Osteoarthritis refers to the wear and tear of the joints and affects one in five Americans.

- ◆ Maintaining your ideal body weight, exercising, and protecting your joints are all important if you have arthritis.

- ◆ Treatment for arthritis can include acetominophen, anti-inflammatory medication, narcotic medication, and joint injections; joint replacement surgery may be an option, if all else fails.

Chapter 16

Hormones and Longevity

In This Chapter

- ◆ Essential hormones
- ◆ Hormone replacement therapy and menopause
- ◆ Options for hormone replacement
- ◆ Manopause and testosterone
- ◆ DHEA, melatonin, and growth hormone (GH)
- ◆ New technologies

The anti-aging movement in the United States really promotes hormone replacement therapy, especially as we hit middle age. Until recently, it was felt that many hormone replacement regimens were completely safe, but more recent data suggests that while there may be some benefit, there is also some risk. In this chapter, we'll look at some of the most common hormones prescribed, along with their risks and benefits.

Some Hormone Basics

Hormones are essential chemicals in the body that stimulate multiple metabolic processes. After being secreted by various glands and tissues, they enter the bloodstream and travel to distant parts of the body, where they exert their effects on just about every biological process in the body.

def•i•ni•tion

From the Greek root *hormo*, meaning to activate or set in motion, **hormones** are chemical substances produced in the body that control and regulate the activity of certain cells or organs. **DHEA** is the abbreviation for dehydroepiandrosterone, a steroid hormone produced by the adrenal glands. It acts on the body much like testosterone and is converted into testosterone and estrogen.

Multiple glands in the body produce hormones, including the thyroid, parathyroid, pancreas, adrenal, ovaries, and testicles, just to name a few. The many hormones produced include thyroid hormone, cortisol, insulin, estrogen, progesterone, and *DHEA*.

As we get older, some levels of hormones, such as estrogen and testosterone, naturally decline. Sometimes our glands may stop producing hormones altogether or fail to produce enough to sustain life. This may happen to the thyroid gland of some adults as they get older, and thyroid hormone replacement becomes essential for survival.

Apart from these essential hormones—thyroid hormone or insulin, if you are a diabetic—scientists have been trying to determine which hormones, if any, might help to reduce disease and disability, or even increase longevity, if given as supplements as we age. While some intriguing pieces of evidence have emerged, there is no fountain of youth hormone that will increase longevity and vitality and not produce any harm.

A Class Act

As you'll discover, hormones perform some important physiologic functions, and understanding them can get complicated. Hormones can be divided into several classes:

◆ *Pituitary hormones:* Produced by the pituitary gland in the brain. They include growth hormone; thyroid stimulating hormone (TSH), which signals the thyroid hormone to do its job; adrenal gland stimulating hormone; and FSH and LH, the hormones that drive sex hormone production in the ovaries in women and testicles in men.

◆ *Thyroid hormones:* Produced by the thyroid gland in the neck.

◆ *Pancreatic hormones:* Insulin and glucagon.

◆ *Adrenal gland hormones:* Cortisol and aldosterone; the adrenals also are capable of producing sex hormones.

◆ *Sex hormones:* Generally produced in the ovaries and testicles, these include a cascade of several hormones all originating from molecules of cholesterol. Cholesterol is converted into pregnenolone and progesterone, which is then converted into DHEA. Finally, DHEA is converted into testosterone and then estrogen. DHEA and testosterone, also known as androgens, affect your sex drive, muscle mass, and bone strength, and women have these androgens just like men, only in lower amounts.

◆ *Adipose tissue (a.k.a. fat):* Your fat cells, primarily those in your belly, are also capable of making hormones and a multitude of other chemicals. For example, estrogen is manufactured in fat cells. Obese people have higher circulating levels of estrogen and are also at higher risk of estrogen-driven cancers, such as breast and prostate cancer.

The American Academy of Anti-Aging Medicine

The American Academy of Anti-Aging Medicine, also known as A4M, was formed in 1992 by Dr. Robert Goldman and Dr. Ronald Klatz. Its members advocate for the use of multiple hormones, especially human growth hormone, and other products purported to reduce the effects of aging and increase longevity.

The A4M now boasts at least 18,000 members in 85 countries and has extensive educational materials and training programs for health professionals. While it has been very good at bringing the issue of aging and the possibility of vibrant longevity to the public, it advocates the use of multiple supplements and hormones, which are not only expensive but also of unproven value in terms of their ability to truly extend health span and life span. In addition, it's important to keep in mind that the anti-aging field is lucrative—the public spends billions of dollars on these products, and physicians and other practitioners who prescribe these remedies often make large amounts of money from their sales. Here's what the research has to say.

> **Doctors' Orders**
>
> The American Academy of Anti-Aging Medicine is not recognized by the American Board of Medical Specialties, and its scientific credibility is questioned by biogerentologists, or those scientists who are considered to be the experts on aging.

Taking a Closer Look

The research does show that you can enhance health and compress or reduce the number of years spent grappling with debilitating diseases, such as heart disease and arthritis. This is achieved *primarily* by avoiding toxins and maintaining those practices that enhance health—healthy diet, lots of varied physical activities, and engagement with life.

What is less clear is whether you can also reverse aging in healthy seniors by plying them with hormones and other supplements. In fact, many well-respected researchers would tell you that this is unlikely if not impossible because of nature's inherent commitment to prolongation of our species through reproduction, coupled with her disinterest in the further increase of life span. In other words, once you've reproduced and passed your genes on, you have fulfilled your genetic imperative of passing on your DNA, and nature probably doesn't much care at that point if you live to be 150 or older.

The Ramifications

Still, there remain some important questions. Do you really *want* to live to be 150 or older, especially if a significant portion of those years might be spent in less than robust health? Furthermore, can our planet even sustain a population that continues to age and survive and consume resources? *Biogerontologists*, the scientists who search for new ways to keep people youthful and to prolong life, must grapple with these ethical and moral questions.

def•i•ni•tion

Biogerontology is a field of geriatrics dedicated to the study of the biological changes associated with aging. Some researchers in this field, known as biomedical gerontologists, also hope to discover ways to extend life and prevent or even reverse aging. They feel that humans are probably capable of living 150 years or longer, given the right circumstances.

Estrogen: Elixir of Youth?

So back to the initial question: will hormone therapy keep you healthy and increase your longevity? Many health practitioners in the anti-aging movement advocate for lots of different hormone supplements as you get older, including estrogen, progesterone, testosterone, DHEA, and growth hormone. Will they really make you feel like you're 25 again and make you live to 100? There's only minimal data on all of this thus far, but we'll review what's known right now. Let's start with estrogen.

We used to think that hormone replacement for women after menopause was a wonder drug—reducing your risk of heart attack, stroke, dementia, frail bones, and probably increasing your life span as well. Our suppositions, however, were based on faulty data. A little hormone history is in order here.

Longevity Facts _____

Lest you think that ovaries produce only estrogen, think again. Ovaries produce two estrogens (estradiol and estrone—and estrone can then be converted to the third female estrogen, which is estriol). The ovary also produces progesterone, testosterone, and androstenedione.

Symptoms of Menopause

Symptoms of *menopause* are many and varied. Vasomotor symptoms include hot flashes, flushing, and night sweats. (Up to 85 percent of women in the United States have vasomotor symptoms.) Genito-urinary symptoms include vaginal dryness, painful intercourse, and bladder and/or vaginal infections.

Other symptoms commonly reported by women in midlife:

◆ Insomnia

◆ Mood swings, irritability, anxiety, depression

◆ Fatigue, forgetfulness

◆ Headache and backache

◆ Stiffness, soreness

◆ Diminished libido

◆ Urinary incontinence

◆ Palpitations

def•i•ni•tion _____

Menopause is the cessation ("pause") of the menstrual cycle for one year or more. The average age of menopause in the United States is 51 years. (The range is 40 to 58 years.)

Managing Menopause Scientifically

The search for hormonal treatments for the symptoms of menopause first began in the 1800s. It wasn't until the 1920s and 1930s, however, that researchers began to isolate estrogen compounds from the urine of pregnant women, cattle, and horses.

The first estrogen replacement product was marketed in the United States in 1933 and was called Emmenin, an estrogen isolated from the urine of pregnant women. Researchers continued to work in the animal realm, however, because this was cheaper than using human sources. The Wyeth-Ayerst pharmaceutical firm subsequently began producing an estrogen compound from the urine of pregnant mares and named it Premarin. In 1942, Premarin was approved by the FDA to treat menopausal symptoms.

The Rise of Premarin

In the 1950s and 1960s, use of Premarin to treat menopausal symptoms became widespread. In the mid-1960s, sales really took off when Dr. Robert Wilson published first an article in *Newsweek* and later a book titled *Feminine Forever*, promoting Premarin as an elixir of youth, guaranteed to reverse the ravages of aging in women and restore them to their feminine youthfulness. He stated:

"A woman's body is the key to her fate. Her fulfillment depends on one crucial test: her ability to attract a suitable male and hold his interest over many years.

The transformation of a formerly pleasant, energetic woman into a dull-minded but sharp-tongued caricature of her former self is one of the saddest human spectacles. The suffering is not hers alone—it involves her entire family, her business associates, her neighborhood storekeepers, and all others with whom she comes into contact. Multiplied by millions, she is a focus of bitterness and discontent in the whole fabric of our civilization."

And thus women began taking Premarin, not only because it reduced the hot flashes, sweats, and other uncomfortable symptoms of menopause, but also because they were promised it would reverse aging, keep them youthful, and keep their spouses from wandering.

Disturbing Developments

Premarin became one of the top-selling drugs in the country; between 1963 and 1966, its use grew about 170 percent. Then around 1980, it was discovered that Premarin given just by itself to women with a uterus increased their risk of uterine cancer. Sales dropped off sharply but then rebounded when progesterone added to Premarin was found to prevent most cases of uterine cancer.

Around that time, studies looking at populations of women taking hormones suggested that hormone therapy might not only treat the symptoms of menopause, but also reduce the future risk of heart disease, stroke, dementia, and osteoporosis. Thus, sales of hormone therapies started a steady climb again. Then in 2001, data from the Women's Health Initiative (WHI) began to suggest that hormone therapy, at least when given to older women, not only did *not prevent* diseases of aging, but actually *increased* a woman's chance of heart disease, stroke, blood clots, dementia, and breast cancer. So that elixir of youth *was* too good to be true.

A Small Silver Lining

The latest data emerging from the WHI suggests that hormone therapy is probably safe when given to younger women—those women in the early menopause, especially those who would benefit because of significant hot flashes, sweats, and other menopausal symptoms. In fact, if used during the early menopausal years (ages 50 to 59), estrogen even seems to reduce mortality from all causes by about 30 percent—a sure way to increase your longevity!

This experience with estrogen has been highly educational for many physicians and scientists, as they try to sort out what other hormones and treatments might reduce symptoms, increase vitality and well-being, and perhaps even increase longevity as we age. Until there are good studies showing not only that these treatments are beneficial, but also that they do no harm, it's important to be cautious.

Words to the Wise

Primum non nocere—the Latin phrase taught to all medical students in the beginning of their training—translates to "First do no harm," and cautions those dispensing medical advice and treatments to be as certain as possible that what they are recommending will not cause harm to the patient. Physicians would be wise to keep this in mind before advocating the use of inadequately tested hormones and other anti-aging treatments.

To Replace or Not—That Is the Question!

Why take hormone replacement therapy at the time of menopause? We have already seen that it does not seem to reduce the risk of chronic disease or increase longevity, and it may indeed cause harm. However, estrogen is better than any other alternative therapy for the reduction of the troubling menopausal symptoms of frequent hot flashes, night sweats, vaginal dryness, and insomnia. Estrogen therapy reduces these symptoms in over 80 percent of the women who use it.

Other things can also help with these symptoms. Regular vigorous exercise is probably helpful, as are calming therapies—meditation, yoga, and paced breathing. Avoiding alcohol and spicy foods may also help. If you are doing everything that you can in your lifestyle to minimize symptoms and you are still uncomfortably symptomatic, then a trial of hormone therapy may be indicated. Fortunately, there are many options available now, including very low dose therapies.

There are other benefits to estrogen. The WHI did show that estrogen therapy can strengthen bones and reduce fractures; it may also reduce the risk of colon cancer. These benefits can certainly add to your longevity, as long as the risks do not cancel them out.

These days, the consensus is that if you don't need hormones, don't take them; however, for menopausal women with troubling symptoms, estrogen replacement can be a godsend.

Types of Hormone Replacement for Women

If you do use estrogen for menopausal symptoms, fortunately there are now many options available, including multiple forms of delivery, as well as low dose preparations.

There are also multiple types of estrogen. Premarin, the form that is made from the urine of pregnant mares, is still popular. Many women prefer more natural types of hormones, including estradiol and estrone. Many women also take testosterone for that droopy sex drive; we'll discuss that in more detail in a few pages. But first, let's look at the controversy over bio-identical hormones, also known as natural hormones.

The Bio-Identical Dilemma

While the WHI put the kibosh on the indiscriminate use of Premarin after menopause, this large and costly study did not look at the health impact of other types of estrogens, such as estradiol, which is the form of estrogen naturally made by our ovaries. The WHI also did not look at natural forms of progesterone, nor did it examine the impact of testosterone replacement on women's health and longevity.

Because of the concern over Premarin, many companies started touting the benefits of *bio-identical hormones.* Look at just about any publication or product for menopause today and you will see these products advertised big time, with claims that they will not cause any harm or increased risk of disease because they are *identical* to the natural female hormones. This is misleading, and the record needs to be set straight.

def•i•ni•tion

Bio-identical hormones are those hormone products that are chemically identical to those made in the ovaries. They include estradiol, estrone, estriol, progesterone, and testosterone. All of these natural hormones are actually made in a laboratory, just as Premarin is.

Most studies were done with Premarin because Premarin was the first estrogen product developed for use in menopausal women in the 1940s and also because the manufacturer, Wyeth-Ayerst, provided it free to researchers. It's only been in the relatively recent past that scientists have been able to manufacture "natural" hormones—i.e., hormones that are identical to those produced in the human ovary and adrenal gland (just as we synthesize insulin for diabetics that is identical to the insulin produced in the pancreas). Most of these products are manufactured from progesterone, which is synthesized from diosgenin, a chemical found in soybeans and wild yams. The point is that none of this is completely "natural"—there's a lot of lab work going on here!

Many practitioners in the alternative medicine field tell their female clients that these natural hormones are completely safe because they are identical to the hormones made by humans. *However—and this is a BIG "however"*—keep in mind that hormones are hormones—and *any* hormone that you take, natural or not, has the potential (albeit small) to increase your risk of cancer and other medical problems.

There are no good scientific studies looking at the long-term safety of bio-identical hormones in terms of cancer, heart disease, stroke, or dementia. Given the recent data from the WHI, we have to assume that *any* hormone, natural or not, has the capacity to cause more harm than good when taken long term. One might even say that the only truly natural menopause is one navigated without hormone pills. Nature obviously did not intend for women to be exposed to any hormone pills after menopause, or she would have equipped the ovaries to do so. Due in part to these concerns, in January 2008, the FDA sent warning letters to pharmacies that prepare bio-identical hormones, expressing concern about their claims.

That said, an integrative approach will combine your healthy lifestyle strategies with hormones *when needed*, so:

◆ Take care of yourself—daily exercise, stress management, and healthy diet do make a difference as you move through the menopause.

◆ Avoid alcohol and spicy foods, which can make hot flashes worse.

◆ Wear layered clothing that can easily be removed if you do get hot.

◆ Use the power of your mind—reframe your hot flashes as "energy surges." Tell yourself they will pass and use paced breathing to reduce your symptoms. Up to 50 percent of women taking placebos in menopausal studies get better. That tells you that if you believe something will help you, it often does!

If you still feel miserable, can't sleep because you're sweating, flashing, and your moods are all over the map, then by all means discuss hormone therapy with your doctor. Take the lowest dose that relieves your symptoms and try to wean off in 6 to 12 months.

Progesterone

Progesterone is used in the hormone replacement cocktail to prevent endometrial cancer in women who have a uterus. There are several synthetic forms of progesterone available; Provera is one of them, and this is the form that was used in the WHI study. Natural progesterone, until recently, was not absorbed if taken by mouth, but now oral forms are available. If you do take a progesterone, choose natural progesterone over the synthetic varieties, as it does not adversely affect your lipids as much as the synthetic varieties can.

Midlife and Hormones: Men Included

Because nature always tries to balance things out, it also created a menopause for men. Just as estrogen and progesterone levels drop off in women after menopause, testosterone levels also begin to fall in men (and women, too) in their 40s, and many men and women also note a drop in their libido. Men may also have trouble achieving and maintaining an erection (erectile dysfunction or ED), and women may note difficulty with sexual arousal or achieving orgasm, especially if they have had their ovaries removed.

Testosterone supplements have become more popular in the recent past, in part because of several books written by well-known personalities that laud the benefits of this hormone. While it may not make you feel like you're 21 again, testosterone supplementation in both men and women with low blood levels may help to restore healthy sexual functioning. It may also improve bone strength.

There are risks to using testosterone. Testosterone may raise blood cholesterol levels and may increase the risk of heart disease. And once again, long-term studies are unavailable, but there's that ever-present concern about cancer risk, especially hormonally affected cancers such as breast and prostate.

DHEA

DHEA is a hormone produced mainly in the adrenal glands and in the testicles in men. It is a precursor molecule to both androgens and estrogens and is one of the most abundant hormones in the body. It also tends to drop off as we age, though exercise will raise blood levels.

DHEA is another hormone supplement that is touted by the anti-aging movement. Short-term studies have suggested that DHEA may improve aging skin, bone strength, menopausal symptoms, and erectile dysfunction, especially if blood levels are low. Some data also suggests that mortality in men, in particular, is increased if DHEA levels are low in men under the age of 70. However, it is not known if DHEA supplementation will increase longevity. In addition, because DHEA can be converted to sex hormones such as estrogen and testosterone, there is concern that persistent use of this hormone can also increase the risk of cancer.

Melatonin

Melatonin, a hormone produced by the pineal gland in the brain, is also used to promote longevity. There is not much data to support this use, but it can help to reduce insomnia, especially in older folks. It has also been used for patients with several different types of cancer, including cancers of the breast, prostate, colon, lung, and stomach; it may help to improve tumor regression and thus increase longevity.

Melatonin can cause drowsiness; you should not drive or operate machinery for four to five hours after taking it. It is also not known whether melatonin supplements can suppress the normal secretion of this hormone from the brain.

> **Doctors' Orders** _____
>
> The purity of these over-the-counter hormone supplements is always a concern, especially if they might have been obtained from an animal brain. If you decide to try melatonin, you should look for a product synthesized in the lab. Often, a compounding pharmacist will be able to specially prepare a hormone supplement for you; however, keep in mind that compounded drugs are not regulated by the FDA and have occasionally been found to be unreliable in their purity.

Hormone Testing

Many alternative health practitioners advocate the use of saliva tests to measure hormone levels in the body. The results of these tests are then used to formulate a specific hormone prescription for the individual. Saliva tests are not covered by most health insurance plans, and to have them done by an independent lab usually costs at least a couple of hundred dollars. Are they worth it? Do they provide better information than hormone blood tests? The answer is probably no. Keep in mind that most hormones are secreted in a pulsatile fashion, so trying to measure the level of a hormone at one moment in time doesn't tell you the full story of how much of that hormone is secreted throughout the day or week.

Growth Hormone

Growth hormone (GH) is produced by the pituitary gland located in the brain. It is needed for normal growth and development; a deficiency of this hormone in childhood results in dwarfism. An excess in childhood results in gigantism, while an excess in adults causes a condition called acromegaly, resulting in an enlarged head, hands, and feet. All of these conditions are fairly rare. With normal aging, blood levels of GH do tend to drop, as do many other hormones. Growth hormone also falls with obesity.

Growth hormone was not available as a safe medical treatment for those with deficiencies until the mid-1980s, when scientists learned how to make it in the laboratory. It is currently only available as an injectable medicine.

In 1990, a small study published in the *New England Journal of Medicine* looked at the effect of GH treatment on 21 normal men over the age of 60. The men received injections of either GH or a placebo three times per week for six months. At the end of the study, Dr. Daniel Rudman and his colleagues found that the men who had received the GH had lower body fat, more lean muscle, and denser bones.

This one small study was enough to prod a group of ingenious doctors to popularize GH treatments as the cure for aging, and the American Academy of Anti-Aging, as mentioned earlier, was born in 1992. More studies have been done since then, but none of them long-term, so we really have no good data on the long-term benefits or risks of ongoing GH treatments. Also, as soon as you stop taking GH, the benefits disappear, so you need to take it continuously to maintain the changes.

Risks and Benefits

In otherwise healthy adults, the benefits of growth hormone use are not clear-cut. A recent article in the *Annals of Internal Medicine* reviewed what was felt to be the best of the studies on the use of GH in healthy older adults. The people in these studies were treated for about 27 weeks; they lost on average 4.5 pounds of fat and gained about 4.5 pounds of muscle. There was no significant change in serum cholesterol levels or bone density.

People getting growth hormone did, however, have a significantly higher risk of soft tissue swelling, joint pain, and carpal tunnel syndrome. They were also more likely to develop elevated blood sugar and diabetes. There is also some concern that inappropriate use of growth hormone may increase the risk of certain cancers. Other studies have found no improvement in muscle strength, endurance, or thinking ability in people getting growth hormone. Studies in mice suggest that GH actually *shortens* survival.

Worth the Expense?

Using growth hormone definitely has a negative effect on one's wallet, as do many of these expensive alternative treatments. Growth hormone must be injected in order to work; it may be given once daily or several times per week (although the human pituitary secretes GH every 90 minutes or so, so even one injection a day doesn't really mimic what our bodies normally do).

The average daily dose is approximately 1 unit. The cost can range from $8 to $18 or more *per unit*, setting you back up to $10,000 or more per year, especially if you have to pay a physician to provide it for you. Some people do obtain it over the Internet and self-administer at home. It's important to note that the use of growth hormone to prevent aging has not been approved by the FDA, and it is currently illegal to distribute growth hormone as an anti-aging substance in the United States.

If you stop to think what kind of vacation you could take for that kind of money or, better yet, what kind of personal trainer or chef you could hire to whip you into optimal shape, you might decide these strategies are far more likely to increase your health and longevity than growth hormone. Besides, as soon as you stop taking GH, all those 4 pounds of muscle you've built up disappear, just like your vacation. Contrary to popular notion, currently available GH supplement pills cannot be absorbed from the GI tract; in fact, many "growth hormone" pills contain no growth hormone at all.

So, if GH injections are not recommended, what else can you do? Fortunately, there are things you can do to maximize your GH function and secretion as you get older—all for a lot less money than a hormone supplement:

- Get enough sleep; growth hormone is secreted primarily at night while you sleep, and sleep deprivation reduces this.

- Take steps to reduce stress in your life; chronic stress also reduces GH secretion.

- Maintain your weight; GH levels drop with obesity.

- Be sure you get enough healthy protein in your diet; this may also stimulate GH release.

- Be sure to get weight-bearing exercise; this will build up muscle just as well as GH.

Growth Hormone Releasers

As we've noted, human growth hormone cannot be taken orally; it is destroyed in the stomach. That's why GH must be taken by injection. There are many companies, especially on the Internet, that try to sell growth hormone releaser pills, including some amino acid supplements. None of these has yet been proven to increase the release or blood levels of growth hormone. Save your money.

The Future: Stem Cells, Gene Technologies, Nanotechnology, and the Like

We certainly have fooled Mother Nature in the past, and, while hormones may not be the answer to increasing your longevity, newer technologies of the future such as stem cell interventions, *nanotechnology*, and genetic treatments may do just that.

def•i•ni•tion

Nanotechnology is a multidisciplinary new field of science that is developing technologies and treatments on a minute scale. As in the 1966 film *Fantastic Voyage,* nanotechnologists may one day be able to treat human beings with tiny atomic or molecular-sized tools or medications that specifically target unhealthy tissues. To give you an idea of the scale of this technology, one nanometer is *one-billionth* of a meter.

Many promising new therapies are being developed, which will probably cure disease, may possibly alter cell aging, and may increase health span and life span. Our idea of what's possible today in terms of longevity may be completely turned upside down by tomorrow's innovations.

These therapies will most likely supplant the need for many hormone treatments currently in vogue.

The Least You Need to Know

 ◆ Hormone replacement can be life-enhancing and even life-saving to those who truly need it, such as people with inadequate insulin or thyroid hormone.

 ◆ Hormone replacement with estrogen and progesterone is no longer recommended routinely for all menopausal women; its risks are felt to outweigh its benefits, and it may shorten life span.

 ◆ Hormone therapy with sex hormones such as estrogen, testosterone, and DHEA may improve quality of life for some; its use should be monitored by a physician.

 ◆ Growth hormone has not been shown to increase health span or life span in otherwise healthy older adults and is also associated with a number of risks. It is also hugely expensive.

 ◆ New technologies such as gene therapies and stem cell treatments will probably make many hormone therapies obsolete.

Chapter 17

Look Younger, Feel Younger

In This Chapter

- ◆ Your skin's life is in your hands
- ◆ Cosmetics conundrum
- ◆ Dermatologic procedures
- ◆ Considering plastic surgery

Does looking better necessarily make you feel healthier? It just might. Looking younger can be associated with a sense of well-being. Some people may feel that a youthful appearance helps them maintain an edge in the competitive business world. Others may use it to attract or keep their mates.

Dermatology (from Greek *derma*, "skin") is a branch of medicine dealing with the skin and its appendages (hair, nails, and sweat glands). A dermatologist is a medical doctor who specializes in this area. The cosmetic dermatology industry is huge, and there are thousands of products and promotions on the market. Plastic and cosmetic surgeries and procedures are also more popular than ever for aging baby boomers. Learn which ones are worth your money and which you might want to leave on the shelves.

Protection Is Primary

Protecting your skin and preventing damage is definitely preferable to having to resort to damage control. If you want to keep your skin smooth and supple for as long as possible, there are two essentials to keep in mind: avoid excessive exposure to the sun and don't smoke. Smoking damages your skin's collagen and elastin, the fibers that give your skin its strength and elasticity. When these fibers are damaged, your skin sags and wrinkles prematurely. Smoking ages your skin rapidly and adds years to your face.

Protection from UVB and UVA Rays

*UVB*s (the "burning" rays) are short-wave solar rays and are extremely potent in producing sunburn. Exposure to these rays can contribute to the development of three different types of skin cancer: basal cell, squamous cell, and melanoma. More than 1 million new cases of skin cancer are diagnosed every year. According to the American Academy of Dermatology, nearly half of all new cancers are skin cancers. *UVA*s (the "aging" rays) are long-wave solar rays and are less likely to cause sunburn but can enhance UVB's cancer-causing effects, especially of melanoma skin cancer. UVA rays also penetrate the skin more deeply and are a chief cause of wrinkling and leathering of the skin.

Doctors' Orders

Stay away from tanning beds! These are not safe alternatives to sun exposure.

Currently, most sunscreens have more UVB protection than UVA protection. The SPF, or sun protection factor, is a term used around the world to designate the ability of a sunscreen to block UVB waves—multiple ingredients in sunscreens are approved for this purpose. The American Academy of Dermatology recommends that you use a sunscreen with a minimum SPF of 15 to protect yourself against UVB waves.

Blocking UVA waves is a bit trickier, and not all products on the market that claim to protect against UVA really block the deepest and most harmful UVA waves. Avobenzone is the only currently available ingredient that blocks these deep waves, but it can break down in the sun. Helioplex is a patented sunscreen formulation that contains avobenzone plus other ingredients that stabilize it. It is probably the best product on the market to protect against UVA; it also blocks UVB rays. To ensure the best protection from UVA, the American Academy of Dermatology now recommends you look for a product containing avobenzone (also known as Parsol 1789), ecamsule (also known as Mexoryl SX), zinc oxide, or titanium dioxide.

The term "water-resistant sunscreen" usually means that the product will protect you for about 80 minutes in water, so remember to reapply it after swimming—or better yet, swim with a "rash guard" shirt.

How much sunscreen should you put on? Think "shot glass" when applying sunscreen. Most of us apply too little. We need one ounce (the equivalent of one shot glass) full of sunscreen when applying it to the entire body.

SPF Explained

The SPF of a sunscreen indicates the length of time a person can be exposed to sunlight before getting sunburn with protection compared to how long the skin takes to redden without protection. As we've mentioned, the current recommendation is that people use a sunscreen with an SPF of at least 15. Those with darker skin may use a sunscreen with an SPF of 6 to 8.

Your clothes can also protect your skin against the damaging effects of the sun; the thicker the weave on the clothes you wear, the better the sun protection. Cotton clothes have an SPF around 4 and cotton/poly blends can provide an SPF of 11.

While your clothes can help protect you, your car windows won't! Studies have shown American drivers have more photodamage (damage to the skin from the sun's rays) on the left side, and Australians have more photodamage on the right. UV protectant film applied to your car windows can help.

Sunscreens may give you a false sense of security, causing you to stay in the sun longer than you normally would. The best way to avoid skin cancer is to not only use a broad spectrum sunscreen but also avoid excessive exposure to the strong midday sun (10 A.M.–4 P.M.), wear a hat, and wear sun-protectant clothing. Sunscreen, however, remains an effective way of reducing sun damage when applied liberally and frequently (every two hours).

Doctors' Orders

Watch out for the skin condition that can kill! A mole that is irregular in color or shape, is changing in size, has uneven borders, has varying pigmentation, or is bleeding should be examined by a dermatologist to determine if it is a malignant melanoma. A melanoma is the most serious and life-threatening form of skin cancer. The dermatologist may biopsy the suspicious mole. If it is malignant, it will be excised in the dermatologist's office and sent for pathology review.

What's in Your Cosmetics?

Over the course of the last century, thousands of chemicals have been introduced into our environment. While some of these are known toxins (some, such as DDT and CFCs, were subsequently banned), many of these have not been studied thoroughly for their safety. There are a number of chemicals that have been used in cosmetics; these include phthalates, parabens, and metals such as aluminum (used in deodorants).

Chemicals Galore

Phthalates are "plasticizers," and help to soften normally rigid plastics such as PVCs. Phthalates are found in multiple products, including cosmetics, clothing, pharmaceuticals, nutritional supplements, medical devices such as IV tubing, and children's toys.

Phthalates, along with other substances such as DDT, PCBs, dioxin, and heavy metals, are known as endocrine disruptors because they exert hormonelike effects on endocrine tissues, including the thyroid gland, breasts, ovaries, and testes. Some data has suggested that phthalates affect fertility and reproductive organ development in both animals and humans.

The European Union has banned the use of phthalates in cosmetics; however, it should be understood that the level of exposure in most products is very small, and the data about harm in humans is preliminary.

Organic Alternatives

Organic and natural cosmetics offer alternatives to cosmetics that include potentially hazardous substances. Per USDA guidelines, at least 95 percent of the ingredients in any food, food product, or cosmetic must be organic in order for that product to qualify for the "USDA Organic" seal.

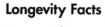

Longevity Facts _____

Organic does not necessarily mean gentle when it comes to your skin, and natural doesn't necessarily mean good for you. It simply means "occurring in nature." Peppermint can irritate the skin and coconut oil can clog your pores. Always read labels and become an informed consumer. Look for the USDA Organic seal on your food and cosmetics where possible. More information is available at www.ams.usda.gov/nop.

Many companies that manufacture natural beauty products have joined the Campaign for Safe Cosmetics, which advocates removing from cosmetics any ingredients suspected of being a carcinogen, mutagen, or reproductive toxin. Check out the Organic Consumers Association online (www.organicconsumers.org). This is a grassroots, nonprofit organization committed to food and environmental safety.

Improving Outward Appearances

Perhaps in a perfect world, we would not be concerned about our outward appearance and accept without complaint what nature has given us. However, the reality is that a majority of consumers are *very* concerned about their appearance in regard to aging. A 2006 Harris Interactive consumer survey of 800 women ages 35 to 69 showed that the majority would like their face to look about 13 years younger. (No surprise there!) Women in the survey were also likely to be extremely or very concerned about the physical appearance of their skin in terms of wrinkles and sagging skin.

Concern about outward physical appearance has led to increased spending on cosmetic procedures—topical, injectable, and surgical. Quick and easy procedures have escalated in use, as consumers find they can easily fit these into their lifestyle. More than two and a half million chemical peels and wrinkle injections (Botox and similar procedures) were done in 2000, and the top dermatologic procedures of 2006 included Botox, chemical peels, laser hair removal, hyaluronic acid treatments, and microdermabrasion.

Botox

Botox injection is currently the most common dermatologic procedure. Botox is made from botulinum A toxin, a purified protein made from botulism bacteria. Botox temporarily paralyzes nerves in the areas where it is injected so they cannot contract and cause wrinkles. It smoothes wrinkles in the neck and face to create a slightly more youthful appearance. It can be especially useful in the forehead and on crow's-feet around the eyes. It is also frequently used around the mouth and in other areas, such as along the chin and jaw.

Botox may also be helpful in treating migraine headaches, certain muscular disorders, and disorders of excessive sweating of the palms and underarms. Side effects from Botox can include a skin rash, allergic reactions, and weakness of adjacent muscles. Injections last about four months and need to be repeated to maintain the desired effects.

Chemical Peels

The second most common dermatologic procedure is a chemical peel. A chemical peel consists of a chemical solution applied to the skin to burn off the outer layers. The skin that emerges from this is smoother, with fewer fine wrinkles and fewer pigmentation changes.

There are three basic categories of chemical peels, varying from gentle to strong. Each type works differently and produces different results. The stronger the chemical peel, the deeper and the more impressive the results. However, the deeper the peel, the more pain you're likely to experience and the longer the recovery time will be.

◆ Light peels use alphahydroxy acids (AHAs) and betahydroxy acids (BHAs). Light peels are the mildest of the chemical peels and can include glycolic, lactic, and fruit acid peels (AHA) or salicylic acid (BHA). They burn off the skin's outer layers and may need to be repeated to achieve the desired result. Light peels are effective for treating fine lines on the face. These peels are generally performed in the doctor's office and take about 15 minutes—hence their nickname, "lunch-hour" peels.

◆ Medium peels use trichloroacetic acids (TCA). This is generally used to treat skin with moderate sun damage, surface wrinkles, and uneven skin or pigment abnormalities. TCA peels are performed in the doctor's office or outpatient surgery center.

◆ Deep peels use phenol acid. Phenol acid is the strongest chemical peel solution. Phenol peels are used to treat skin with deeper wrinkles and blotchiness. Phenol peels can be done in a doctor's office or outpatient surgery center.

These peels cause significant swelling and some pain and require some recovery after surgery.

Laser Hair Removal

Hair, hair everywhere—especially where you don't want it! You pluck one and two grow back. How do you remove hair permanently? Electrolysis is a traditional semi-permanent method that cauterizes and destroys each individual hair follicle. Some hair may need repeat treatment later on. The laser procedure can be time-consuming and somewhat painful, but the pain is less than with electrolysis. Laser hair removal is a growing trend in hair removal and the third most common elective dermatologic procedure.

The laser works by sending energy into the pigment of the hair shaft. The energy is absorbed by the surrounding hair follicle. The heat generated by the laser damages the follicle and stops hair production, thus effectively removing hair from the unwanted area. This procedure works best for those with dark hair and light skin tones.

Longevity Facts

Many types of lasers can also be used to rejuvenate the skin. Some of these lasers act on the deeper layers of the skin, while others are relatively superficial, for faster recovery. Broken blood vessels, brown spots, and superficial wrinkling can be improved with many of these devices.

Hyaluronic Acid Injections

Hyaluronic acid has been approved by the FDA as a "skin filler," which decreases the appearance of fine lines and wrinkles and is usually used in the face. It is a naturally occurring component of the skin and works by holding together collagen and elastin, which provide a framework for the skin. Hyaluronic acid can be used with collagen for an optimal cosmetic effect.

Hyaluronic acid is injected into the skin in a gel form; it binds to water and provides volume that fills in large folds of skin (such as those around the mouth and cheeks). Hyaluronic acid gel does not pose an allergy risk for patients, and results last approximately four to six months. The injections can be painful (so usually some type of numbing agent is used) and produce temporary swelling and redness—especially in the lip area.

Microdermabrasion

Microdermabrasion is a process that removes the dead outer surface of the skin (stratum corneum). This is done with mechanical abrasion through a handheld wand, using particles such as zinc oxide or aluminum oxide crystals that rub against the skin. Microdermabrasion also stimulates the production of skin cells and collagen.

Microdermabrasion is effective with superficial skin conditions such as early photo-aging (result of sun damage to the skin), fine lines, and superficial scarring. It can be used to soften the appearance of crow's-feet, age spots, and acne scars. Each treatment takes from 30 minutes to an hour; it can be mildly painful.

Plastic Surgery Quick Fixes

What used to stay up inevitably falls down, and we all eventually see wrinkles, bags, and sags where firm skin used to be. This is in part due to natural aging and loss of elasticity in the skin. It is also due to lifestyle factors, such as sun exposure and smoking.

The American Society of Plastic Surgeons estimates that in 2006, 11 million cosmetic procedures were performed in the United States, and 1.9 million of these were surgical cosmetic procedures. There has been a 55 percent increase in breast augmentation since 2000, but a 22 percent reduction in the number of facelifts. However, there are still a large number of people undergoing facelifts and eyelid lifts. In the over-55 age group, around 115,000 people underwent eyelid surgery and around 67,000 underwent a facelift.

> **Longevity Facts**
>
> The word *plastic* in plastic surgery derives from the Greek *plastikos*—meaning to mold or to shape—which is what plastic surgeons do to the body. It does not refer to the synthetic plastic.

Based on statistics from the American Society of Plastic Surgeons, the top surgical procedures of 2006 included breast augmentation, rhinoplasty ("nose job"), liposuction, eyelid surgery, and tummy tucks.

It's not surprising that lifting various parts of the body has become a sought-after surgery for the over-40 crowd. In fact, this age group had a 12 percent increase in lifting procedures (thigh lifts, lower *body lifts*, upper arm lifts, breast lifts, tummy tucks, and face lifts) from 2005 to 2006. Divided up by gender, women account for over 90 percent of all cosmetic surgery procedures performed in the United States.

def•i•ni•tion

> A **body lift** is a surgical procedure that removes excess fat and skin and improves the appearance of cellulite or dimpling in the skin. A body lift may include:
> - Abdominal area—either front or around the sides and into the lower back
> - Buttocks that may be droopy, uneven, or flat
> - Groin area that may sag into the inner thigh
> - Thigh—including the inner, outer, or posterior thigh, or circumferentially (all around)
> - Arms—usually the flabby skin under the upper arm

Why Choose Cosmetic Surgery?

The reasons for choosing to have cosmetic surgery are myriad and personal. It could be for reconstructive purposes—either because of a birth defect or to repair the result of trauma or injury. Plastic surgery may also be done to slow the aging process or to correct a feature a person never liked, such as a big nose or a receding chin. Others have plastic surgery to stay competitive in their jobs or in response to comments about their wrinkles, such as "You always look tired or angry."

There is generally no single right reason to have surgery, but there are many wrong ones:

◆ "My husband/wife left me." New relationships or failed old ones, a job loss, or a midlife crisis are not good reasons to have surgery.

◆ "I've always had low self-esteem." Split-second decisions are generally not good where plastic surgery is involved. Elective surgery should be well thought out.

◆ "I am depressed and the surgery will help." Patients with active mental disorders—untreated depression or anxiety—should get these conditions treated prior to seeking surgery.

◆ "I've never liked the way I look—I want to look like someone else." Drastically changing your features is not what surgery should be used for; instead, it should enhance what you have. Patients with a history of multiple surgeries to achieve perfection may be looking for something unattainable.

Cosmetic surgery is not to be taken lightly. It involves significant expenditure of your time, money, and emotions. It comes with a potential risk of surgical complications. Be aware of what your motivations are in choosing surgery prior to deciding to get it done.

Reducing Complications from Plastic Surgery

The risks with plastic surgery include the potential risks of general anesthesia (for those procedures that cannot be done with injectable anesthetics). Specific risks for particular procedures include blood loss, infection, skin loss, asymmetry, slow healing, scarring, numbness, and minor dimples and puckers.

A 2004 study in the journal *Plastic and Reconstructive Surgery* found that serious complications from tummy tucks, breast enlargement or reduction, liposuction, and other cosmetic surgeries were rare—but they did occur. The rate of serious complications was 0.34 percent and death was 0.0019 percent.

You can reduce your risk of surgical complications by doing the following:

- Verify your surgeon's credentials. Cosmetic surgery is best performed by a physician who has gone through training to perform certain types of cosmetic procedures. Depending on the procedure involved, this could be a plastic surgeon; a facial-plastic reconstructive surgeon; or, in some cases, a dermatologic surgeon who has received training for the procedure in question.

- If you are undergoing plastic surgery, this is best performed by a physician who has gone through training to be a plastic surgeon and received board certification in Plastic Surgery. This would include completing at least five years of surgical residency training, usually three years of general surgery, and two years of plastic surgery.

- Educate yourself about your procedure: the risks and benefits, the recovery time, and any side effects or potential complications. (See Chapter 3 for more on recovering from surgery in general.)

Health Benefits of Cosmetic Surgery

Whereas there is no data that shows that people who have cosmetic surgery live longer, there is certainly data showing that an enhanced sense of self-image can lead to many health benefits. Studies suggest that patients who are pleased with the outcome of their cosmetic surgery report improvement in self-esteem, social confidence, and quality of life.

A strong self-image can lead to changes in how you deal with others. You may become more confident and more effective in your work relationships. You may have an improved sense of well-being and be more comfortable in your intimate relationships.

Words to the Wise

Cosmetic surgery is not a quick fix for poor self-esteem, self-confidence issues, or relationship problems. Counseling should be the first step to resolve those issues. But in individuals with a healthy emotional life, plastic surgery can be the icing on the cake.

Breast Implant Health Risks

There have been several long-term studies on breast implants, and some prior fears about implants do not appear to be valid. There is no reproducible link to increased breast cancer or autoimmune disease in women with saline breast implants. There is, however, a significant link to an increased rate of depression and suicide in women who have implants.

Recent data from a large Canadian study tracked almost 25,000 women who received breast implants between 1974 and 1989. The study showed a 75 percent increased risk of suicide in women who had implants versus a control group. The number of suicides were small overall but were statistically significant.

Other studies have also found increased risks of depression, lower self-esteem, and *body dysmorphic disorder* in women who have had implants. It is not that the implants cause suicide or depression, but rather that some people who opt for the surgery may actually have unrecognized or untreated psychiatric issues.

If you feel depressed or have low self-esteem, you should get this evaluated and treated by your doctor or mental health provider prior to embarking on implants or any other cosmetic surgery procedure.

def•i•ni•tion

The Mayo Clinic defines **body dysmorphic disorder** as a condition in which individuals have a distorted or exaggerated view of their appearance and become obsessed with their physical characteristics or perceived flaws.

The Least You Need to Know

- The best way to keep your skin looking youthful is to avoid damage from smoking or sun exposure.

- Certain chemicals present in cosmetics, including phthalates, may be harmful to the body; natural cosmetics are an alternative.

- Dermatologic procedures commonly used to erase the effects of time include Botox, skin peels, and micordermabrasion.

- Cosmetic surgery is becoming increasingly popular in older populations, and there are both right and wrong reasons to have this kind of surgery.

- Data shows that an improved self-image leads to improved relationships and improved emotional health.

Part 4

Passion for Life: The Ultimate Longevity Booster

Study after study has found that people who are optimistic, have deep social connections, and have love and spiritual fulfillment live healthier and live longer. They fare better after heart attacks, have less dementia, and have lower rates of depression. So how do you fill a prescription for a full and balanced emotional life? Where do you even begin? This part provides what you need to know in the field of mind-body-spirit medicine to help you tap into the wellness it can offer.

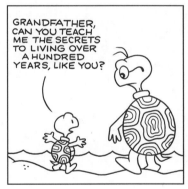

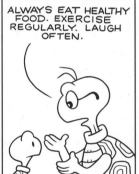

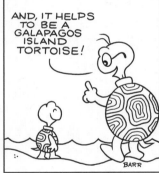

Chapter 18

Unlocking the Power and the Potential of Your Mind

In This Chapter

◆ An emerging field of medicine

◆ Using your thoughts to reframe your life

◆ Relaxation techniques

◆ Becoming your own life's hero

◆ Write it down to let it out

◆ Visualizing health

Not long ago, scientists thought of the mind and the body as two separate entities. They didn't believe the brain exerted much influence on the body. The brain was felt to be the *generator* of mind and consciousness and not the other way around. Science didn't consider that the mind could influence the brain or our state of health, or that changing our thoughts might shift our moods and our physical well-being. Although it is still not clear what it is that actually generates consciousness, modern medicine is discovering that the mind has the potential to significantly improve overall health and well-being and probably increase longevity as well.

Mind-Body Medicine: Psychoneuroimmunology

The field of mind-body medicine, known as psychoneuroimmunology, is a relatively new one. This is a long word, and one that's packed with meaning: *psych* refers to the mind, *neuro* to the brain/spinal cord/nerves, and *immunology* to the immune system. This emerging science is exploring the mind's intricate relation to the workings of the body and vice versa.

Until the 1970s, conventional scientific wisdom held that the mind had little to no influence on the body. Serendipitous discoveries in research at that time, however, served to open up a whole new world of possibilities for healing and led to glimpses of the body-mind as one integral system of intelligence, conveying information back and forth in a seamless dance of information. Scientists learned that the cells of the brain/nerve, immune, endocrine, and gastrointestinal systems literally talked to one another in a constant flow of information in the form of chemical messengers called neuropeptides or *neurotransmitters*.

def•i•ni•tion

A **neurotransmitter** is a chemical messenger released by a cell that travels to a nearby or distant cell to relay information. Once thought to only be produced by neurons (cells of the nervous system), neurotransmitters have been found to be produced and also received by nearly every tissue in the body.

This field of research has since exploded. We are now looking at how interventions in some of these areas can have a positive impact on illness, life span, and health span. What does this mean for you and me? Futurists, those folks who envision what lies ahead for us all, predict that the future of medicine will be primarily focused on the power that we have to impact and change our bodies, brains, and minds through focused intention and attention. If this comes to pass, you will be able to harness the power of your mind and your body to create phenomenal well-being in your life. In *no way* is this an indictment of someone suffering with an illness. Rather, this emerging science offers us an opportunity to address what is needed to restore balance in our lives.

The Stress Factor

We now know that chronic and uncontrolled *stress* has a negative impact on the immune system and other body tissues. In fact, it is estimated that anywhere from 50 to 80 percent or more of the physical symptoms that bring people into the doctor's office involve stress-related mind states, including anxiety, worry, and depression. We also know that if people learn to experience themselves as helpless and hopeless when confronted with stress, their immune system is more likely to function poorly. When this happens, illness and infections are more likely to occur. Chronic, unremitting stress has been found to lead to or aggravate a number of medical conditions, including heart disease, irritable bowel syndrome, heartburn, insomnia, depression, infertility, and chronic pain.

Can relaxation techniques help to prevent or reduce these conditions? The answer is yes, though we are still investigating the power of meditation and other relaxation techniques to impact disease. You'll read more about this later in the chapter.

def•i•ni•tion

> **Stress** is a condition of mental, emotional, or physical upset or strain that generally produces chemical and physical changes in the body, including an outpouring of adrenaline, increased muscle tension, and elevated heart rate and blood pressure. While stress can be a normal part of our physiology, chronic unhealthy levels of stress can eventually harm the body.

Thinking About Thoughts

Thoughts constantly pop up unbidden in our minds; we are so inundated by them that we're not even aware of them most of the time. If you try emptying your mind of thought, you will find it nearly impossible. You may find yourself saying, *I'm not having any thoughts*, but that in itself is a thought.

Emotions, on the other hand, are the feeling states that arise when we assign meaning to our thoughts or to situations or events. For example, if someone cuts you off on the freeway and you focus on the thought, *That should not have happened—what a jerk!*, chances are you will soon experience the emotion of anger. Emotions result in the production of chemicals and neurotransmitters in the brain, and these substances then produce changes in the body. Persistently negative thoughts and emotions will often lead to anxiety and depression.

Reconsidering Illness

Illness and physical symptoms tend to capture our attention; they offer us an opportunity to wake up and address imbalance in our lives. Many people report that illness was one of the best things that happened to them, because it put them on a healing pilgrimage they otherwise might not have taken. For example, a heart attack might make you realize that you're not going to live forever; it might get you to change your diet, exercise more, and stop smoking. It might also inspire you to quit that job you hate and start going after what's really important to you. This is often referred to as authentic self-expression: the expression or assertion of one's own truth or true nature. We find ourselves awake and enlivened. Who could ask for a better longevity formula?

Bolstering the Immune System

Authentic self-expression can support and strengthen our immune systems and may facilitate healing; this is being tested in human research. For example, a recent study showed that gay men who are HIV positive and out of the closet are less likely to experience disease progression than men who conceal their homosexuality. Another study of non-HIV-positive gay men showed that those who were still in the closet were almost three times as likely to develop cancer, as well as infectious diseases, as those men who were open about their sexual orientation.

Longevity Facts

Studies looking at the impact of humor and laughter found positive changes in immune cells of participants in the study. Cultivate your sense of humor and you may live longer!

There are numerous other studies looking at how mind-body techniques can positively impact the immune system. For example, it has been shown that the process of writing (telling the truth) about difficult or painful past memories improves immune function and overall health. Lab tests in these studies confirm protective changes in the immune cells of the participants. Bottling up or shoving aside painful emotions, however, seems to adversely affect our immune cells.

Other fascinating research findings include the following:

◆ The placebo response, long the bane of clinical researchers, suggests that those who take a sugar pill in a research study often get the same benefit as those people taking the drug under study. It seems that our *belief* in something has the power to change us physically as much as a real drug.

◆ People with a suppressed history of physical or sexual abuse are more likely to suffer from chronic intestinal or pelvic complaints, including irritable bowel syndrome and chronic pelvic pain.

◆ Dr. John Sarno, a pain expert at New York University, has had great success in helping his patients heal from chronic neck and back pain by having them identify and then release long-repressed emotions, especially anger and rage.

The Plastic Brain

We used to think that once brain development was complete, the brain was rigid, i.e., unchangeable. Recent studies show that the brain is a lot more malleable than once thought, and with a little brain-training, we may be able to reach new heights in our quest for healing.

Neuro-plasticity suggests that the brain and the mind are not fixed or static, but in fact are capable of changing, remodeling, or even growing, given the appropriate circumstances. Brain cells connect with each other through their physical connections and also through neurotransmitters. This mass of connections tends to reflect our mental focus—our thinking patterns. If we learn new tasks or if we start to change the focus of our thoughts, this will also start to change some of the connections in the brain, and we may even change the brain tissue itself. The good news is that we can all learn to do this through practice, persistence, and intentionality.

Relearning Thinking

Cognitive behavioral therapy (CBT) is a relatively new form of psychotherapy used to treat anxiety and depression. It teaches us to challenge our negative thinking with more realistic assessments of ourselves and the situations in which we find ourselves. Rather than focusing on fixing ourselves or our past, CBT looks at what is creating suffering for us in the present moment. Cognitive therapy also helps us to identify what we wish to create in our body-mind and focus our attention on that.

Buddhist mindfulness meditation teaches a similar approach. Both cognitive therapy and mindfulness meditation employ techniques that teach us to stop identifying with and attaching to our dysfunctional thoughts and to step back and simply observe them as they pass by, in much the way clouds pass by in the sky. Once you step back from attaching to your painful thoughts and instead become simply the observer, they begin to lose their hold on you. You might even find that they disappear just as randomly as they appeared. You learn how to *have* your thoughts without letting them have control over you. If you do this training in a group, you also learn that everyone has dysfunctional thoughts, and you stop taking them personally.

Truth vs. Perception

These two concepts are hugely important in mind-body medicine. An example: if you took 100 people and put them all through the same experience, such as being in a car accident, you would come up with 100 different interpretations or perceptions of what was true about that situation. Some of those people might have perceived the situation to have been extraordinarily stressful; others might have ruffled nary a feather, but each one would probably be certain that his or her interpretation was the *right* one.

The *truth* is that the motor vehicle accident happened; the interpretation, which is always personal, is how each individual *perceives* the situation. Our perceptions are molded by the ways we learned to interpret the world when we were children, and many of us learned to interpret the world as a fearful place, especially if we faced abuse or serious trauma in childhood. Fortunately, we can learn to change our perceptions. This, in simple terms, is where the power of cognitive therapy comes in.

> ### Words to the Wise
>
> To paraphrase Albert Einstein: the most important question any of us can ask ourselves is "Is it a friendly universe or not?"

Cognitive behavioral therapy teaches us to come up with different perceptions and interpretations for our experiences, especially for those that have been difficult for us or have led to chronic symptoms, including anxiety and depression. We can learn to create new interpretations that are life-enhancing and that leave us empowered, rather than trapped.

Meditation and Relaxation

While we are all familiar with the stress response in the body—the physical changes we experience when we are frightened by something and feel the effects of the outpouring of adrenaline—some of us have never experienced the power that we have to cultivate the opposite response. *Meditation* and other relaxation techniques provide a means to achieve this. Herbert Benson, M.D., a pioneer in stress research at Harvard University, coined the term the Relaxation Response in his book of the same name (see Appendix B) to describe the physical changes that occur in the body when we meditate or practice other relaxation techniques.

def•i•ni•tion

> **Meditation** is an ancient practice of stilling the incessant activity of the mind, usually by focusing on the breath, on an object, or on a word. This focus brings us into the present moment, rather than allowing our thoughts to carry us off into the past or future. Meditation is usually done when one is sitting or lying down but can also be done while walking. Meditation leads to physiological changes and relaxation, even if one lacks the perception that anything has changed in the body.

In the 1990s, Dr. Jeffrey Schwartz at UCLA showed, in a small study of patients with moderate to severe obsessive-compulsive disorder (an extreme form of anxiety), that 10 weeks of mindfulness meditation training not only improved patients' symptoms but also reduced the activity in the brain associated with this type of anxiety. This was the first study to show that a mind-body approach, such as meditation, was capable of changing brain chemistry; numerous other studies have since validated this approach.

Dr. Jon Kabat-Zinn, another pioneer in this field, developed a patient program at the University of Massachusetts called the Mindfulness-Based Stress and Pain Reduction Program (MBSR). This 10-week course combines mindfulness meditation with yoga and journaling. It has been enormously successful in helping people reduce stress, depression, and chronic pain and is now offered at medical institutions throughout the country. Dr. Kabat-Zinn's program has also been shown to improve immune function. His program is described in his book *Full Catastrophe Living* (see Appendix B).

You are not the anxious or depressed person you *think* you are; you may, however, be someone who has become habituated to this. As the saying goes, "Change your thinking, change your life." While medications for anxiety and depression can be a godsend, these consciousness-raising practices can be a helpful adjunct to your treatment protocol.

There are practices other than meditation that can also produce the Relaxation Response in the body. These include guided imagery, visualization, self-hypnosis, and progressive muscle relaxation. When you cultivate the Relaxation Response in your body, your blood pressure decreases, your heart rate comes down, your breathing slows, and your muscles relax.

The secret to all of this, of course, is practice and persistence. Most of us are already quite skilled in latching on to negative thoughts. Daily practice of meditation and focused intention, however, can train your brain cells to fire in different directions and to make new connections. You can train your mind to move to the positive.

Meditation and observation help you shift from "Mindful-Mess" to "Mindful-Ness"—a place where you can relax and give yourself a break. This is also the space where new ideas and new possibilities are generated. Once you add a little intentionality here, you're on your way to generating what you want for yourself and your life, instead of running on that negative autopilot.

What Lies Between Your Ears—Friend or Foe?

It is estimated that 95 percent of our thoughts are recycled; the same repetitive stuff cycles through our brains over and over. For most of us, the constant noise that rattles around in our heads is not our best cheerleader. Our inner critic is often the most active thing going between our ears, and most of the stuff we're battered with is a bunch of recycled failures from the past or worries about what will probably never happen in the future.

If you're someone who has ever experienced depression or has a tendency toward pessimism, you can relate to this. Some anthropologists think that we may be hardwired for a little pessimism and worry; after all, if our early ancestors hadn't had a little apprehension for what dangers might be lurking around the corner, they might have ended up as some animal's dinner. The key here is awareness. You may respond automatically to events with that glass-half-empty approach, but with a little cultivated awareness, you can learn to put that thought on hold and trade in your hard-driving inner critic for a cheerleader.

Longevity Facts

Studies of Buddhist monks who are adept at compassion-based meditation show significant enhancement in the parts of their brains that generate empathy and love. Recent studies have shown that these changes in the brain even seem to motivate people to take compassionate action in the world. Related to all of this is the concept of *attention* and *intention:* what we pay attention to and focus our intention on does in fact literally change the brain and may lead to change in our outward behavior as well.

Reframing Your Life and Your Stories

Ever notice that the world seems to be made up of stories? We all have a story to tell about who we are, where we come from, and why we turned out the way we did. Who doesn't love a good story—and the juicier, the better! Some of us have had idyllic pasts, filled with loving friends and family and lots of success. Most people in the world, however, have had to navigate some pretty tough stuff through childhood and into adulthood.

This may mean that what you bring into your adult life is a fixed idea of what you are and are not capable of and how safe the world is, but this is not who you truly are!

Your family life and your childhood circumstances, your neighborhood/city/country, and your culture have given you a background. Now *you* get to take all of that to the next level. You get to be the hero of your own journey.

Consider that you are the storyteller, the myth-maker for your village. You are entrusted with writing stories that will be handed down to the children and grand-children of the village. Remember that all heroes face seemingly insurmountable odds, struggle with dragons or other fearsome beasts, get lost in dark forests with no road maps, and face the loneliness of abandonment. Your task is to write your story from the hero's perspective. If you were this hero, how would you tell your story? Describe how your hero faced difficult situations; dealt with despair, hopelessness, and failure; and turned them into newfound strengths and lessons. What gifts have come your way out of what you have grappled with? What lessons would you want to pass on to the children yet to come in your family? What ancestral wisdom will you leave them with?

In looking at your life in this way, you can begin to move beyond being the victim of unforeseen circumstances to the hero who has faced the obstacles put in his or her path and used them as a means to become authentic, strong, and whole on this journey.

Writing Your Way to Wellness

Writing can be a powerful way to have a positive effect on your immune system and your physical well-being. A number of studies have been done looking at the power of writing as a means to disclose or release difficult, painful, or shameful emotions. Bottling up what's painful can keep it hidden from the outside world for a while, but you can't escape its impact on your inner workings, including your immune system.

Writing with Intention

You may say, *I don't repress my stuff—I talk about it all the time, especially to my friends, but that doesn't seem to help.* Here's where a little intention may help; consider writing or disclosing the tough stuff with the intention of releasing it—letting go and moving on.

For some of us, what's difficult has become familiar; it's become part of our story, it's who we know ourselves to be. Giving that up might indeed be a little scary. You may find yourself asking, *If I don't have chronic pain, will my family still be there for me?* or *If I'm not the disabled one, if I get better and even lose my disability income, then where will I be and who will take care of me? Will I be able to take care of myself?*

These can be challenges to releasing illness and physical symptoms and getting well again. If you find yourself in this space, consider getting some professional support.

Writing to Release and Heal

Choose something to write about that has been stressful for you; perhaps an unresolved trauma from childhood that was significant for you. Avoid recent traumas, or anything that may be too upsetting for you right now.

Find a quiet place where you will not be disturbed for at least 20 minutes. Write for 20 minutes about the event, including any thoughts or feelings you have about it. Do not edit your work; just write in a stream of consciousness style. Do this for three to four days in a row. Daily journaling may be even more beneficial.

> **Longevity Facts**
>
> A 1999 study of people with both asthma and rheumatoid arthritis showed that writing about painful experiences for 20 minutes a day three days in a row resulted in significant improvement in both physical symptoms and also in measurement of disease activity. This study, published in the *Journal of the American Medical Association*, was the first to show that writing about difficult experiences actually improved the objective measurements of disease by the patients' doctors.

Another Approach

Tell your story from another's perspective. For example, if your stressful tale involves unresolved issues with your mother, try writing from your mother's perspective. What was her world like when she was born? What struggles and injustices did she have to overcome as she was growing up? How must it have been for her when her mother died? What were her strengths, her weaknesses, and her disappointments? What gifts did she bring into your life? Putting yourself into another's world can help you gain a broader understanding of the fabric of your family's and friends' lives. This will reduce your perception of stress, your levels of stress hormones, and potentially your risk of getting sick. Healing brings health, and health brings long life.

The Power of Intention

If our thoughts do have the capacity to alter our physiology, then perhaps with a little focused intention we can engage this practice in creating better health for ourselves.

Perhaps, as some new thought physicists and philosophers suggest, our lives don't look the way we want because we're putting more attention on what we *don't* want than on what we'd really love to have for ourselves. We may have more power than we've given ourselves credit for to create the life we want.

> **Words to the Wise**
>
> There are two ways to live: you can live as if nothing is a miracle; you can live as if everything is a miracle.
>
> —Albert Einstein, physicist

The Treasure Map

Every great invention or outcome in history began as a thought or as a seed of an idea in someone's consciousness. You can begin to transform your thoughts into physical reality by first creating what some have called a Treasure Map—this is intention at its best. Sit quietly for 10 to 20 minutes and focus on a particular goal or desired outcome. Imagine it as vividly as you can—if it is an object, visualize its size, shape, color, smell, location, etc. If it's something less tangible, such as a trip you've always wanted to take, then imagine where you will be, what you'll be doing, etc. If your goal is a health outcome, such as healing from back pain or depression, then visualize your body regaining vibrant health and see your mind being peaceful and wise. Bring in as much detail as you can. It also helps to write down the date that you intend to make this happen—make it time-based and measurable.

Then, go through your favorite magazines and cut out pictures or words that call to you about your visualization. Arrange the images and words into a collage on a poster board or piece of paper. Hang this up in a place where you will see it every day. When doubt arises, as it inevitably does, go back and refocus on your collage, holding your intended goal in mind. Let it also inform you of the actions you will need to take to achieve this goal.

Guided Imagery as a Healing Tool

Imagery is the language of the intuitive—of creative ideas, dreams, fantasies, and grand plans and also of fears and worries. Our minds work primarily in imagery, even though we may often be unaware of it. Images provide a window to the intuitive, to our inner wisdom, that we often don't hear because of the constant distraction in our external world.

Imagery has the capacity to produce physiological changes in the body, including changes in the autonomic or *involuntary* nervous system (for example, your body temperature or heart rate). A simple example of this is what happens when you imagine that you are licking a slice of a sour lemon: as you imagine what it tastes like, your mouth and your taste buds react as if you are actually eating the lemon. Another great example is what happens in the body when you worry about an upcoming event, such as taking a final exam. Imagining a dire outcome produces physiological changes in the body, including the release of adrenaline and other stress hormones from the adrenal glands, which produce increased heart rate and muscle tension and all of the other physical outcomes of the fight-or-flight response.

> **Words to the Wise**
>
> Change the way you look at things, and the things you look at change.
> —Wayne Dyer, Ph.D., author and lecturer

The Healing Within

Imagery has been used for healing for many decades, but it is only in the past few decades that it has been used and studied in earnest for the relief of emotional and physical pain and illness. Many studies now confirm the power imagery has to alter stressful physiological responses and help people heal. In some ways, imagery is also akin to hypnosis. Both of these techniques can be learned and practiced individually or under the guidance of a trained practitioner.

Using Imagery

There are several different ways in which imagery is used. Imagery can be used simply to help reach a state of deep relaxation to initiate the Relaxation Response. Imagery can be used in two other ways, however, when used with the intention of healing a physical symptom or condition. In evocative imagery, we try to evoke or elicit an understanding or insight about the symptom or disease and why it might have shown up in the first place. For example, someone with chronic shoulder pain may see that their pain represents an experience of being burdened, or having to shoulder a lot of responsibility. In directive imagery, one uses imagery with positive suggestion to direct inner healing forces to heal the illness. Both evocative and directive imagery are often done, or guided, with the help of a therapist trained in these techniques, hence they are referred to as *guided imagery*.

Imagery can also be used to evoke what is needed to motivate and sustain health-inducing actions and behaviors. As an example, a patient with chronic hand pain of unknown origin realized that her pain was the only thing she felt safe talking to her mother about; it was a means for them to stay connected. When she was able to see this and develop more empowered ways of communication, her pain lessened and almost resolved.

Guided imagery is now used in many hospitals to reduce the pain and anxiety that accompany illness and surgical procedures. Studies have shown that guided imagery can help reduce the amount of pain medicine needed after surgery and may also improve healing outcomes and reduce the length of hospital stays.

Going for the Image

What do you do if you want to give imagery a try? You can find someone, such as a therapist, who is trained in doing imagery with clients. You can also easily start on your own by purchasing tapes or CDs with imagery scripts. These are especially useful when you are trying to reduce stress in your body-mind. In order for this to be effective, most practitioners recommend that you practice your imagery for at least 10 to 15 minutes, once or twice a day. See Appendix B for resources.

A Quick Start to Evocative Guided Imagery

Find a comfortable and quiet place where you can sit or lie down undisturbed for at least 30 minutes. Begin by focusing on your breath and taking several slow, deep breaths. Keep your in-breath and out-breath even, allowing five to six seconds for each. As you breathe, imagine that, with each in-breath, you are giving space to your thoughts, feelings, and physical sensations. Try to allow everything to just *be*, without having to change or push anything away. With each out-breath, feel your body relax a little bit more.

Now move your attention to a part of your body that has been painful—for example, your lower back. Breathe in and out into your back for a few moments. Then, ask your back to reveal to you the source of its pain. When you listen for answers, you must listen broadly; the answer might come in words, but it might also come in an image, sound, or sensation. You also might not get an immediate answer the first time you do this.

When you feel complete with this, then gradually bring yourself back to ordinary awareness, slowly moving your arms and legs. When you are fully awake, notice what has shifted in your body from this exercise. Write down any insights that might have arisen. If you are not aware of any, then stay open to anything that might reveal itself to you as you go about your day.

Feisty and Fearless/Ornery and Outrageous

After all this talk about doing the right things to create good mind-body health, we can all come up with examples of people who did everything *wrong* (smoke, drink, party all night) and still live to be 90. Could there be something to being a renegade that is life- and health-enhancing?

Webster's dictionary defines a *renegade* as someone who rejects conventional wisdom. There is much we don't understand about why some people get sick and others don't. But perhaps those people who are just willing to be who they are without worrying what others think—people who grab the life they want with gusto and don't let go—do more to generate life force than people who do everything *right*.

This is still a subject of inquiry in medicine, but fearless, outrageous people may be tapping into a life force the rest of us could learn from. Where have *you* been afraid to show the world what you're really made of? Perhaps you will find some healing for yourself in that arena.

The Least You Need to Know

- Your mind and body are intricately connected, and your mind has a greater influence on your health than you may think.

- You can train your mind to think in new directions; this will in turn create changes in your brain and your body.

- Meditation and other forms of relaxation can reduce stress hormones and positively impact your health.

- Rewriting your "story" from the hero's perspective can help you put stressful events behind you.

- Intention is powerful—choose what you want for yourself and see yourself achieving it in the future.

Chapter 19

The Power of Optimism, Hope, and Laughter

In This Chapter

- ◆ Laughter is serious medicine
- ◆ Working past pain and illness
- ◆ Don't take yourself so seriously
- ◆ Seeking joy in your life
- ◆ The practice of Laughter Yoga
- ◆ Changing your life focus

The joys of a blissful mind! Opening your life to laughter has a profound experience on your overall health and can dramatically improve your quality and quantity of life. Can you learn how to be optimistic and happy? Of course you can! Optimistic people get so much more out of life, and humor is optimism's tool of choice.

The Power of Laughter

Laughter really is the best medicine. The preceding chapters may have gotten you thinking along serious lines, and that was the intent. Now, however, it's time to consider another of longevity's power tools—laughter!

The idea of using laughter and humor for healing has been around since biblical times. Laughter generates joy in the moment, pulls our attention away from what is causing distress and anxiety, and helps us to generate a sense of hope and optimism again. Cultures from the ancient Greeks to Native Americans have recognized the power of humor to help us to heal.

Longevity Facts

In 2002, Americans spent over $17 billion on medicines to treat anxiety and depression. Laughter has health benefits that can enhance quality of life, and it doesn't cost anything!

In the early years of the twentieth century, scientist Walter Cannon began some of the first research on the effects of stress on the body. Hans Selye, his student, furthered his work. These two scientists helped to establish our understanding of the impact of stress on our health. They demonstrated that stress had negative effects on the nervous, endocrine, and immune systems, and that stress could be triggered by pain, exposure to cold, and physical activity, as well as by emotions such as fear and anger.

Cannon and Selye also explored ways in which an organism could reverse the impact of stress on its well-being and reestablish balance after being impacted by stress. As you will see in this chapter, one of the most powerful tools we have for reversing stress may indeed be laughter.

Research Studies That Prove the Point

Medical research has only recently begun to unravel what happens physiologically when we laugh deeply. Not only does laughter take our mind off our troubles, it also has positive effects on our immune systems, muscles, circulation, blood pressure, mood, and pain tolerance. Could there be a better prescription for health and longevity?

Norman Cousins, the beloved former editor of the *Saturday Review* and professor of humanities at UCLA Medical School, was one of the most famous examples of a person who used the power of humor to help himself heal. In his late 50s, he was diagnosed with a painful inflammatory arthritis called ankylosing spondylitis and given a very poor prognosis by his doctors. Determined to get better, he checked himself out of the hospital and into a hotel, where he squirreled himself away with old Marx Brothers movies, *Three Stooges* comedies, and anything else he deemed hysterically funny. From there he proceeded to belly laugh as much as he could.

Cousins reportedly said that he could "laugh twice as hard at half the price" in a hotel room compared to the hospital—at probably a tenth of the price in today's dollars! He found that 10 minutes of hearty laughter resulted in two hours of pain-free sleep.

Although it took a number of months, he eventually cured himself of his arthritis and became a strong and well-known advocate for the use of humor, faith, hope, and love to help people to heal and live longer. While teaching at UCLA Medical School, he witnessed many incidents of the power of the mind to either make people sick, or conversely to help them heal.

> **Words to the Wise**
>
> The art of medicine consists of amusing the patient while nature heals the disease.
>
> —Voltaire, writer and philosopher

Saranne Rothberg was in her 30s when she was diagnosed with an aggressive form of breast cancer; she was in stage 4, a medical diagnosis with a grim prognosis. She remembers reading about Norman Cousins and took on his healing approach. While she experienced a great deal of fear at times, she was also determined to continue to find ways to laugh. She received traditional Western medical treatment for her cancer and combined this with her laughter therapy. The result? She found herself in complete remission from her cancer. Her experience led her to found ComedyCures!, a nonprofit foundation that has become nationally known for its work in lifting the spirits of people with illness, trauma, disability, or depression. She is but one example of many who have used laughter in a therapeutic way to heal.

While the study of laughter and healing is still in its infancy, there are a number of researchers who have done and continue to do some fascinating work. First, let's look at what happens to you physiologically when you laugh.

> **Words to the Wise**
>
> A clown is like an aspirin, only he works twice as fast.
>
> —Groucho Marx, comedian and film star

Laughter and Physiology

Dr. William Fry at Stanford University was one of the first scientists to explore the benefits of laughter on the body. His research on laughter actually began in the 1950s, at a time when many doctors were not very open to these ideas. He and his colleagues eventually showed that hearty laughter reduced the levels of stress hormones in the body, including cortisol and epinephrine.

Chronic stress causes chronic increases in cortisol and epinephrine. These increases have multiple negative effects, including immune system suppression and increased risk of infections. Chronic stress is also felt to increase inflammation, which leads to degenerative disease. If laughter is able to mitigate all of this, it has the potential to protect us from degenerative diseases that shorten our life span.

Laughter and Antibodies

Laughter has also been shown to increase the production of antibodies that can protect us from illness. For example, one study showed that laughter increased the production of *IgA*, which protects us from upper respiratory infections such as colds and influenza. Laughter also increases other antibodies that are protective, such as IgG. The increase in antibodies that occurs after watching 30 to 60 minutes of funny videos can last for 12 hours or more.

def•i•ni•tion

IgA is one of several types of antibodies produced by some of our white blood cells. It is found mainly in body fluids, including saliva and tears, where it helps to fight off bacteria, viruses, and other unwelcome visitors.

In one study, people who scored high on a sense of humor test also had higher levels of IgA when compared to people who scored low on the same test. They also seemed to experience less suppression of their immune cells when faced with stressful events.

Laughter and Immune Cells

Laughter also affects natural killer cells (or NK cells), immune cells that are important in fighting cancer as well as infections. Laughter seems to increase the number and activity of these cells, especially in patients whose NK numbers are lower than normal. In AIDS patients, laughter may increase the number and activity of T helper cells, which are the cells destroyed by the AIDS virus.

How does laughter affect our immune cells? It appears that a positive or happy mood has a strong, positive impact on the immune system and vice versa. A happy mood seems to enhance the responsiveness of the immune system, perhaps by reducing the chronic secretion of stress hormones such as cortisol, which suppresses the immune system. Laughter and mirth are excellent ways to help lift yourself out of that bad humor and get your antibodies and white blood cells working full bore again.

Wounds also seem to heal faster in people with positive emotions, perhaps again because of reduced blood cortisol levels.

Laughter and Internal Organs

Laughter has positive effects on your organ systems as well. It works your muscles, especially your core abdominal muscles, resulting in an aerobic workout. It is estimated that 20 seconds of hearty laughter is equivalent to three minutes of vigorous physical activity. One study suggested that 10 to 15 minutes of vigorous laughter burned about 50 calories. As an added benefit, when you stop laughing, your muscles are more relaxed. Laughter also works your respiratory system, increases respiration, and is felt to help clear the lungs of secretions.

Do you hate to exercise? Try laughing instead, and make it a total body workout—get your face, arms, legs, and belly activated and moving. You will feel your heart and respiratory rates go up, just as you would on a treadmill. Your diaphragm will be engaged, and you will breathe more deeply. Keep it up for several minutes, and you will feel as if you've just run a sprint—exhausted perhaps, but with muscles that are much more relaxed.

Laughter and Your Heart

Laughter also seems to protect the heart. A 1997 study at Loma Linda Medical Center looked at the benefits of laughter in a group of 24 people who had just suffered a heart attack. The patients were divided into two groups. Both groups got their usual medical care from their doctors; one group was also asked to watch a funny video of their choice for 30 minutes every day for a year. At the end of that year, only 20 percent of the patients who had the laughter therapy had had another heart attack, compared to 50 percent of those in the routine care group. They also didn't need as much heart medication, such as nitroglycerin. And there's more—they had lower blood pressure and less risk of heart rhythm problems. The levels of stress hormones in their blood, epinephrine and cortisol, were also lower, and this may have been the factor leading to most of the other benefits.

Doctors' Orders

Think you need to feel good in order to laugh? Think again. Laughing for no reason generally *leads* to feeling good, which precipitates more laughter. It's a grin-win situation!

In a similar vein, another study at Maryland University Medical School in 2000 showed that people with heart disease were only 60 percent as likely to laugh in a variety of situations compared to similar folks without heart disease. These same researchers also showed that laughter increased blood flow in the arms by 22 percent, whereas mental stress reduced blood flow by 35 percent. We know that people who frequently feel hostile and angry are at higher risk of heart disease. They tend to take themselves and their lives very seriously and probably have a hard time finding humor in their lives, especially when things don't go their way. And just in case you see yourself in this description, don't worry—everyone can learn to find humor in life!

Laughter and Pain Reduction

Laughter can also help reduce pain. Norman Cousins experienced this, as we noted earlier. Studies since then have confirmed the power of laughter to both reduce pain and increase pain tolerance in conditions ranging from burns to rheumatoid arthritis.

def•i•ni•tion

Endorphins are morphinelike chemicals produced in the brain that reduce pain and produce a sense of well-being. They are nature's own painkillers.

Why is this? Some speculate that laughter helps to increase *endorphins*, the body's own painkillers, but this has yet to be proven by research.

Laughter may also help by reducing muscle tension. When we tense up our muscles, we also contract the blood vessels in those muscles, and this may lead to reduced blood flow to that area of the body. This is felt to increase the perception of pain. Supporting this theory is data that shows reduced pain in patients who practice meditation and other relaxation techniques that help to relax the muscles (see Chapter 18). Many hospitals now teach mindfulness meditation as a means to help reduce chronic pain and the need for pain medications.

Laughter and Diabetes

One small study looked at the effect of humor on patients with diabetes. The study's participants were all fed the same meal and then watched a serious movie. Following the film, their blood sugars were measured. The next day the intervention was repeated, except that they watched a humorous movie instead. Blood sugar measurements were lower after the funny movie compared to the serious one.

Laughter and optimism may have a positive impact on your cells, but will they increase your overall health or longevity? We haven't yet fully measured the extent to which laughter therapy might reduce illness and increase life span, but data is starting to accumulate here, too. These studies are promising and help to support the many other mind-body techniques that are being widely accepted as important players in the quest for health and increased longevity.

For example, one study that followed people over many years found that optimists were more likely to enjoy better physical health than their pessimistic counterparts. Some studies suggest that cancer patients and AIDS patients with a positive fighting spirit also might survive longer.

One interesting study compared longevity between two groups of people over the age of 65. Those in one group declared their health to be good, despite medical evidence that they were ill; those in the other group were more pessimistic and felt themselves to be in poor health, despite medical evidence that they were healthy. Who lived longer? You guessed it—the happy optimists!

Words to the Wise

If you are a sourpuss or view life through a negative lens, this in no way means you are to blame if you contract an illness. In fact, your disposition may have some strong genetic connection. But try laughter anyway. Laughter is free, easy to do, doesn't require any special equipment, and will reduce your stress and make your feel better in the moment. It makes sense to incorporate laughter on a daily basis as part of your longevity tonic. Try making the biggest sourpuss face you can in the mirror and see how long you can keep a straight, sour face!

Laughter and Depression

Laughter helps us maintain optimism and hope. This is enormously powerful in healing and can also reduce the risk of anxiety and depression, when we are facing illness or other challenges in our lives. Soldiers and POWs in times of war often report that they use humor to help themselves cope and survive. Even Viktor Frankl, the famed Austrian psychiatrist imprisoned in a Nazi prison camp during World War II, reported that humor helped prisoners survive the death camp. Humor can help us to maintain control over our emotional reactivity, keeping depression and anxiety at bay.

Lighten Up!

In *The Art of Possibility* (see Appendix B), Ben and Rosamund Zander tell a story about two prime ministers engaged in a serious meeting. The meeting is constantly being interrupted by agitated staff members of one of the ministers, who admonishes them to "Remember Rule #6." This seems to immediately calm them. The other prime minister is intrigued and asks for the secret of rule #6, to which the first replies: "Rule #6? Don't take yourself so goddamm seriously!" When asked what the other rules were, the first prime minister declared, "There aren't any!"

At some point, you are going to find yourself in a difficult or burdensome situation or conversation. By learning to take yourself and your situation less seriously, you can let go of some of that heaviness and lighten up. Once you do that, you generally will feel de-stressed and lighter. In addition to reducing your stress hormones, this usually creates more possibility for creative problem-solving.

Think about your own health habits. If you've committed to a healthy diet but have just gone off the wagon and binged on a pint of ice cream, what's going to get you back on track more quickly—beating yourself up for failing once again, or glee-fully declaring that you've filled your calcium quota for the day? This doesn't mean you give up on self-responsibility. It's just that taking yourself a little less seriously can reduce the dramatic fallout that often keeps you stuck and sends you back to the refrigerator for consolation.

Seeking Joyful Activities: The Birth of Mirth

So what do you do if you don't feel that you're very funny or that you take yourself way too seriously? Don't worry—studies show that people who find humor in their lives have a lower risk of getting sick than those people who try to be funny. In other words, you don't have to be a stand-up comic to reap the benefits of laughter; you just have to be willing to look for the fun and the funny in life. This is a skill you can cultivate.

A Matter of Style

Figure out what your humor style is. What kinds of comedies, cartoons, and jokes make you laugh? What made you laugh when you were a kid? What sitcoms did you enjoy then? Today? Look for ways to bring that kind of laughter back into your life on a daily basis.

Watch something or listen to something funny every day. You can download humorous CDs onto your iPod for your 24/7 listening pleasure. Consider putting it on first thing in the morning to help you set the mood for the day. Rather than going to see another stressful war movie, go to a comedy club instead.

Keep Good Company

Hang out with a 4-year-old and laugh at what she laughs at. You'll find children are masters at seeing humor everywhere.

With which friends do you laugh the most? Spend time with them *and* start to cultivate more humor with your other friends as well. Surround yourself with people who brighten your day. Be mindful of the happiness that exists around you.

Your Own Self

Find ways to bring humor into your everyday world. Laugh more at yourself. Take yourself less seriously, especially when you're trying to do something *just right*, or when you make a fool of yourself (just think *I Love Lucy* …). This is a great opportunity to lighten up.

Laugh at yourself and the world laughs with you!

> **Doctors' Orders**
>
> Think you can't laugh spontaneously? Try this laughter exercise: start laughing from your belly and keep it up for at least 30 seconds. Don't just chuckle, get your whole body into it—bend over, slap your knees, throw your hands over your head. When you've mastered 30 seconds, go on to a full minute. You may not be able to stop. And keep a tissue nearby, in case you're laughing so hard you cry!

Try these suggestions on for size:

- Show up at work periodically with a clown nose or a Groucho Marx pair of eyeglasses and nose.

- Keep your favorite funny book at your bedside and read it when you first get up in the morning; keep another one at your desk for a midday laugh lift.

- Notice the thoughts that pop into your head when you first get out of bed in the morning. For many of us, they're not pretty—*I'm so tired; when can I get back to bed; I have too much to do today.* Notice these without judgment; instead look into the mirror, throw your arms up over your head, and declare "This is going to be an awesome day!"

- Listen to your favorite energizing music and dance! It's impossible to sing and dance and stay depressed—the two cannot occupy the same space in your mind at the same time.

◆ Learn to avoid the energy drains. News and political commentary getting you down? Limit how much you read or listen to it. Best friend always griping? Learn to channel the conversation to positive topics.

Stop and ask yourself: *Will this really matter tomorrow? Next year? In 10 years?* When you look at the big picture, you can learn to laugh at the little stresses in life.

Laughter Yoga

Laughter Yoga is a style of yoga started in the 1990s by a physician in Mumbai, India, Dr. Madan Kataria, who noticed that many of his patients were stressed and unhappy. He noticed a lack of humor in the city of Mumbai as well. Dr. Kataria began to incorporate laughter into the breathing exercises and yoga postures he did with his patients. This laughter was a natural addition to yoga, because deep laughter causes us to inhale and exhale more fully and to use our breath more fully, which is important in yoga.

Dr. Kataria also emphasized cultivating childlike spontaneity, as well as connecting with other human beings through his yoga exercises. People were encouraged to make eye contact with those they were laughing with, something that many of us avoid in our busy workdays. By structuring laughter into the yoga postures, then moving into deeper laughter, his patients were led first to more spontaneous eruptive laughter and then to all of the benefits seen with laughter, including muscle relaxation and reduced stress and stress hormones. The sessions were ended with relaxation and meditation exercises.

This practice was well received by his patients, and popularity for this yoga style began to spread. Dr. Kataria started his first official laughter club in 1995, and there are now over 5,000 Laughter Yoga clubs in 40 countries around the world. The first Sunday in May is now celebrated by this group as World Laughter Day. The premise is that laughter is like a form of meditation: when we laugh, it is almost impossible to focus on things that are upsetting or worrying us, including other people. The website is www.laughteryoga.org.

Health, Longevity, and Optimism

What about the role of optimism in health? Like laughter, optimism is an important player here. Although it seems some of us are born optimistic and others are always focusing on the negative, optimism can be a learned behavior. There's a good reason for learning to lighten up. A number of studies have shown that optimistic people aren't just more satisfied with their lives; they also live longer.

A Mayo Study

A Mayo Clinic study begun in Minnesota in the 1960s looked at the longevity of over 800 people who self-referred themselves to the clinic. All were given a number of physical and psychological tests when they entered the study. By the year 2000, those who had been identified as optimists had 19 percent greater longevity than the pessimists.

A Harvard Study

Dr. George Vaillant, a Harvard professor and author of *Aging Well* (see Appendix B), has conducted one of the longest-running studies looking at factors that affect healthy aging. Beginning in the 1930s, his team at Harvard has followed a diverse group of men in Boston, ranging from Harvard graduates to inner-city youth. They discovered a group of qualities that seemed to predict robust health in older age, no matter what the initial socioeconomic background of the participants. These traits included altruism, a sense of humor, an ability to keep looking toward the future, and the ability to delay gratification.

Humor and laughter were found to be signs of maturity that helped people cope and avoid premature death from stress-related illnesses. About 95 percent of the men who embraced these traits remained robust in their physical vitality into their old age, compared to only 53 percent of the men without these traits.

> ### Words to the Wise
> A merry heart is like a good medicine.
> —Proverbs 17:22

Two More Studies

A study done in 2000, looking at more than 2,200 Mexican Americans in the southwest United States, showed that positive emotional traits, including happiness, were strong predictors of better health and longevity. Happy people also tended to take better care of themselves, which also contributed to their good health, although this in itself did not account for the improved longevity.

Another study, published in 1983, followed medical students over a period of 25 years and found that those who rated themselves as hostile were about five times as likely to develop heart disease in middle age compared to the least rageful students. Numerous other studies have supported this hostility–heart disease association as well. Hostility is also associated with a higher risk of developing other illnesses, including depression. And while it can be therapeutic to resolve anger and frustration, studies have shown that the venting of anger increases blood pressure for both men and women—not something your heart appreciates.

Learning Optimism

Dr. Martin Seligman, a research psychologist at the University of Pennsylvania, is a pioneer in the field of optimism research and on how optimism impacts mood, anxiety, depression, and longevity. He is one of the founders of the Positive Psychology movement, which has studied the impact of positive emotions on health and well-being. He developed a happiness formula which posits that our enduring experience of happiness is the sum of three ingredients:

1. Our *set* range, or what we biologically inherit from our parents; however, this only accounts for about 50 percent of our happiness.

2. Our life circumstances, which account for about 8 to 15 percent of our happiness.

3. The things we have voluntary control over—our perceptions, interpretations, choices, and actions, which account for about 40 percent of our happiness.

While we can't change our genes and may not always have control over our life circumstances, we have complete freedom to generate that in our life which can have a lasting effect on our happiness. Cultivating our strengths and becoming skilled at certain interventions can have a profound impact on our happiness and also protect us from depression and anxiety. These include the following:

- Practicing gratitude for all of the good in our lives; this takes the pessimistic focus off what we *don't* have.

- Learning to forgive ourselves as well as those who might have harmed us.

- Interpreting life events in a way that leaves us empowered rather than victimized—cognitive therapy at its best!

- Learning to savor life.

♦ Doing things we love, especially those things that make us lose track of time when we are immersed in them.

Many other pioneers in this field are convinced that optimism, hope, and determination play a powerful role in the ability to recover from serious illness and live a full life. Doctors such as Bernie Siegel, O. Carl Simonton, Rachel Remen, Larry Dossey, and many others who have worked with people with cancer and other life-threatening illnesses, are convinced that these qualities play an enormous role in healing. Bernie Siegel calls them his *extraordinary* cancer patients—not extraordinary in the sense that they possess some exotic talent that allows them to heal, but extraordinary in that they have taken the reins full-on in the recovery of their well-being. They are determined to play full out, knowing that each day is precious and that the healing journey itself is the prize, not the final outcome.

Doctors' Orders _____

If you are a recovering pessimist, determined to become a glass-half-full devotee, be forewarned: these concepts are simple but take practice and persistence to build them into the fabric of your being. This is not a quick fix, but with intention and practice you will be rewarded with a level of happiness beyond anything you are likely to ever get in an antidepressant pill.

Permission to Be Happy

Sometimes when we've faced difficult circumstances, such as the death of a loved one, it may be difficult to give ourselves permission to laugh again. We may worry about what others might think if we're mirthful when we *should* be mourning.

In a similar vein, many of us grew up in families where there was not a lot of laughter; laughter might even have been considered inappropriate. For example, if you or your family members grew up during the Great Depression, you may have a well-established family story that life is hard work, something to be taken seriously, and laughter might not have found a place in your home. Many of us have a happiness or laughter ceiling above which we are not comfortable rising. Learning to challenge these old beliefs and take risks in creating new stories for ourselves can help us break through these glass ceilings.

Words to the Wise
Against the assault of laughter, nothing can stand. —Mark Twain, author and humorist

Optimism, hope, love, and laughter are all important components of your longevity lifestyle and are, fortunately, all skills that can be cultivated. Happily, for many people, older age is accompanied by softening and grace—the ability to lighten up; to take things less seriously; to let go of old hurts; to forgive and reconnect with old friends; and most importantly, to savor the small, momentous things in life that bring true joy.

The Least You Need to Know

- Optimism, hope, and happiness play an important role in health and longevity.

- Laughter has multiple, positive effects on the human body, including muscle relaxation, improved circulation, and bolstered immune cells.

- Laughter can be a great way to generate humor and happiness.

- Laughter Yoga is a simple and easy way to bring a laughter practice into your life.

- While happiness is, to some extent, genetically determined, it is also significantly impacted by how we train ourselves to view and appreciate our lives.

- We can all learn to find humor more readily in our lives, especially by taking ourselves less seriously.

20

Staying Motivated and Energized to Change

In This Chapter

- ◆ Six stages to making healthy changes
- ◆ Commit to making a change
- ◆ Put an action plan into place and line up support
- ◆ Harness powerful intentions
- ◆ Focus on your goals—and don't give up!

Being inspired is always easiest at the beginning of a good idea. Human nature being what it is, however, the thrill is too soon gone. So how do you stay inspired, committed, and energized? By learning strategies to keep you focused on your goal of achieving a long and healthy life! In this chapter, you'll learn how to create those strategies, along with specific action steps to put those strategies to work for you. Keep yourself focused *with intention* on your goals and you will increase your longevity potential.

The Six Stages of Change

Dr. James Prochaska, Ph.D., a research psychologist at the University of Rhode Island, helped to revolutionize the field of behavioral change in the 1990s, when he studied people who were trying to quit smoking. Prior to his work, behaviorists and physicians encouraged their patients to *just do it*—just quit griping and take action! However, many people failed with this approach because they were not ready or prepared for action or success.

Prochaska began by studying people who were successful in making behavioral change. From his observations, he identified the stages of change that all people seemed to go through as they worked toward their goals. Over and over, he found that successful people consistently went through six stages. He also found that those who failed typically did so because they either skipped a stage or got stuck in a particular stage without the skills needed to complete that stage and move on. Once he was able to pinpoint the stage in which a person was stuck, he could devise strategies for overcoming previous failures.

> ### Words to the Wise
>
> Always bear in mind that your own resolution to succeed is more important than any other one thing.
>
> —Abraham Lincoln, sixteenth president of the United States

Prochaska's approach was proven to have phenomenal power in helping people break addictive behaviors, including smoking, overeating, recreational drug use, and inactivity. His work is now used all over the world to help people make changes that not only enhance their health and longevity but also increase self-esteem and self-efficacy.

You can spend a great deal of time speculating as to why you're not getting results with your self-improvement projects. If you're truthful with yourself, however, you'll realize the problem is a lack of commitment. If your goal is to lead a longer and healthier life, and you've decided it's time to get serious, then it's time to focus in on the power of intention, attention, and action to get the results you want. Lifestyle changes are in order! It's time to see where you currently stand in the six stages of change and learn how you can move through them and make those healthy changes stick! Here is Dr. Prochaska's list, followed by an in-depth explanation of each:

1. Pre-contemplation
2. Contemplation
3. Preparation
4. Action
5. Maintenance
6. Termination

1. Pre-Contemplation

In this stage, you are not convinced you need to change. You are not convinced that some of your behaviors might be negatively impacting your health span or life span. You have not yet started to formulate any ideas about changing your behavior, and there is no intention to change behavior in the foreseeable future.

How do you move out of this stage and into contemplation? You might start by making a commitment to listen to the advice or coaching that others give you, including your doctors, family members, and friends regarding your health, your well-being, and your success. You might also start by identifying where satisfaction and joy are missing in your life. Most of us want to feel satisfied and happy with who we are and what we're doing, and the desire to expand upon this can move you into the next phase—contemplation.

2. Contemplation

Being in the contemplation phase means you recognize that your current behaviors might be negatively impacting your well-being. You see that change would be beneficial to you, but you're not yet committed to making any changes. Some people can spend weeks or even months in this stage. If this describes you, then it's time for a little more action!

> Mr. Taylor is a 51-year-old businessman, husband, and father who owns his own company. He loves what he does but works long hours and feels he doesn't have time to take care of himself. He has been gaining weight gradually since his 30s, and this year at his annual exam he learns that he is now obese. His cholesterol and blood sugar are abnormal as well. His father died of a heart attack at the age of 55. Mr. Taylor is starting to worry about his own longevity but doesn't see how he will find the time or motivation to change his health habits. He has tried to lose weight several times in the past five years but has always gained it back. Mr. Taylor is in the contemplation phase—a good place to start. He recognizes that change will probably increase his chances of longevity.

Time to Make a List!

What are all the benefits that would come from changing your behavior? How would you feel physically or emotionally if you made changes? Write all these down. For example, "I want to get off these diabetes meds, but I won't be able to unless I exercise and eat better."

Doctors' Orders

Take ownership of your well-being. Just as you get to know people by asking them questions about themselves, ask yourself questions about your goal. Here are some to consider:

♦ How will life look when I reach my goal?

♦ What doors will open up for me if I make changes?

♦ What will my accomplishments with this goal enable me to do next?

This is also a good time to identify the barriers that might stop you from changing your behavior. Common barriers for most people include:

♦ I don't have enough time.

♦ I don't have the money.

♦ I'm too tired.

♦ I don't feel like it; I just don't have any willpower.

Conquering each of these can actually be simple, with a little insight, logic, and planning. Barriers start to disappear as you put more energy on what you want and less energy on why you can't. It's vitally important to focus on finding ways to make your goals happen. You might even find that what you need shows up pretty effortlessly. The willingness to look for solutions is paramount in this stage. Let's address each of these individually:

♦ *Excuse #1: I don't have enough time.* Start by making a list of all of the things you do in your free time, such as watching TV, reading, and hanging out with friends. Set aside some of that time for a new goal, such as exercise. For example, you realize that you could exercise while watching TV and that this could be a great use of your time. You realize that your best friend also wants to get in shape and suggests that you start taking walks together, so you blend your friendships with your exercise—you friendercise!

◆ *Excuse #2: I don't have the money.* This is another common concern (and complaint) of many people, but those who are focused on what they want never let this stand as a permanent obstacle. You can begin by looking at your discretionary money—the money you spend on coffee, lunches, or cosmetics, for example. These quickly add up to lots of cash. Create a well-being account, and set aside money for this every week, instead of that latte. If you want to purchase some home exercise equipment, consider sharing this expense with a friend. You could also look into community programs such as the YMCA, which are much less expensive than many fitness clubs.

◆ *Excuse #3: I'm too tired.* This can be so seductive—it's a great excuse. Yet doing what you love is energizing, and so is exercising and eating a healthy diet. Once you start moving forward, you will have more energy—guaranteed. Chances are, you'll also sleep better. You'll feel more vibrant and alive—the best longevity tonic there is.

◆ *Excuse #4: I don't feel like it; I just don't have any willpower.* This is really saying that you're not committed to that goal. If that's the case, reexamine your goals—come up with something that you really *are* committed to. When you're trying to change behavior, resistance always sneaks in, sometimes in tricky disguises such as boredom, frustration, despair, anger, and fatigue. You don't have to cave in to these, and this is where cheerleaders, coaches, and support people are really helpful. Doing something you promised you would do is the best solution for conquering that willpower monster. Once you start and you complete those first small steps, the mastery will expand your sense of your own power and capacity and lead to the next success. This is the ultimate definition of self-esteem: coming to know yourself as someone who is capable of powerfully declaring and creating what you want in your life.

> **Words to the Wise**
>
> Evaluate your commitment. A commitment to good health, or anything else for that matter, is much easier when it's chosen for yourself and not to please someone else.

Other Barriers to Change

Clean up the distractions in your space. New ideas need room to grow, so clean up the clutter around your living and work space. Clean up your emotional space, too: complete undone tasks, reconnect with the people who are important to you, forgive yourself and others for perceived past failures, and get ready to move forward.

You might also discover some *disadvantages* of going on this journey. Sometimes behavioral changes, even when they seem positive to you, can seem unsettling to those around you. For example, if your spouse has been used to being the breadwinner in your home, and you're now inspired because you're back in school working toward that graduate degree you always dreamed about, this may change the dynamic of your relationship, and your partner may feel threatened. Identifying disadvantages does not mean you throw in the towel; it just shines light on areas in your life you may need to proactively address as you go forward.

3. Preparation

In stage three, you intend to change a behavior and you've begun making a plan for action. Perhaps you've joined a gym or signed up for a class; perhaps you've purchased the equipment you will need, such as walking shoes. Maybe you remember how you longed to dance when you were a teenager, and you've signed up for a dance class. This is also the time to enlist a buddy to support (and perhaps join) you in your new activities. You schedule your exercise times in your day-planner. You start with realistic, achievable goals; for example, starting with a 5- or 10-minute walk every day instead of a 60-minute race. You accept the fact that no one goes from couch potato to Olympic athlete overnight. You start to think about what you will be doing over the next year and how you will progress with your plan. You now also clearly identify what could potentially get in your way, such as your work schedule, and you identify strategies for dealing with setbacks.

> **Doctors' Orders** _____
>
> If you get stuck in the preparation stage, don't worry—it's common! It really helps to sit down with your calendar and your telephone and start to make some specific plans; for example, schedule an exercise appointment and put that in your calendar. Call your exercise buddy to confirm a date. Schedule a time with a fitness trainer. Clear time in your schedule if you need to. And then keep those appointments!

Don't wallow in your history of past failures. Instead, make a list of what you *have* accomplished, even when you doubted that you would. (If you can't think of a single event, here's one for you—you learned to walk, even though the chances of success might have seemed highly implausible to you as a toddler.) Recognize that if you are truly committed to your goal, you'll make this one happen, too.

If you're still feeling a little stuck or overwhelmed, it's probably only a sign of where you've put your attention in the past—on being stuck and worried. Now, however, you're going to put the laser focus instead on your goal—on the prize, on *intention!*

Imagine your life shows up inside the viewfinder of your camera; it looks pretty fixed—as long as your camera is focused on one spot, the picture doesn't seem to ever change. Now imagine you move your camera, and what shows up in the viewfinder is the image of the life you dream of—this is where you will now focus your attention and your energy.

Create Some Quiet Time

If your goal still seems a little fuzzy or unfocused, this might be a good time for some inner work. Reflection, meditation, and visualization are useful tools to help you identify what's really important to you (see Chapter 18). When you create the opportunity to quiet your mind, to lessen the constant barrage of noisy thoughts, then your intuition or your inner voice is easier to hear.

> Mr. Taylor begins the process of changing his behavior. He decides to start with exercise; he wants to get fit again. He remembers how much he used to enjoy cycling when he was in college, and he remembers how good he felt and how much energy he had when he exercised regularly. He makes a list of all the things that he loved about cycling. He also realizes that he could ride his bike to work. Then he remembers how much he has wanted to teach his sons about the joys of cycling, but somehow hasn't found the time. He takes his bike to the shop to get it tuned up and finds that they have family fun rides he can do with his kids. His sons are excited about this new venture with their dad. He is now in the preparation phase.

The Power of Intention

Now that you've connected with what's really important to you, you're ready to formulate goals. Having the clear intention to bring something new into your life is a powerful place to begin a new practice, such as regular exercise. The field of mind-body medicine is rapidly elucidating the power of our thoughts and intentions to bring about desired changes in our lives; following are some tools to help you.

◆ Put your intentions up everywhere as constant reminders of what you're up to in this adventure.

◆ Make a collage of your intended outcome using pictures and words from magazines or other print media. Hang your collage where you'll see it every day.

◆ Clear your space of temptation. Get rid of what tempts you and pulls you away from your goal—from your home, your office, your car, etc. It's hard to lose weight if the pantry is packed with junk food.

◆ Tell everyone what you're up to; allow people to coach you and support you and to hold you accountable to your commitments. Choose your cheerleaders!

◆ Get a calendar and map out your goals and actions. What actions will you take every day and every week to reach your goals?

Watch out for guilt. When you fall off your commitment, guilt can sneak in and make waste of all your good intentions. Allowing yourself to wallow in guilt is really just a way to justify your return to bad habits. Recognize guilt, acknowledge it, and then get back on the horse!

4. Action

This is the stage where you take action—you are in the *doing* phase! This is exhilarating because you're doing what you promised yourself, and you're also starting to notice some benefits. Perhaps you have more energy now that you're exercising on a regular basis. Here it's important to set up your environment so that it supports your success. If you go to the gym to exercise after work, always keep your workout clothes in the car so you're ready to go; have fresh fruit on hand as a snack after your workouts, etc. It's also important to use *positive self-talk* here, to start to identify yourself as the person you are seeking: I am a walker, I am an athlete, etc.

def•i•ni•tion

Positive self-talk is the practice of replacing negative, self-critical thinking with positive, productive affirmations. It involves first recognizing what's getting in your way (the negatives) and then consciously making the effort to turn this pattern around to help you achieve your goals.

The action stage lasts for six months. This is a critical time, as you work toward making your action feel like a normal part of your life, rather than an effort. Positive reinforcement is key in this stage; this is the time to give yourself a healthy reward for your great efforts. This also is where a buddy, a coach, or another support person can help to keep you on track; in fact, fill the bleachers of your cheering section!

The Support Network

Support networks are especially helpful when you're tackling something difficult. Here are some ideas to help you build that network:

◆ Get a buddy! Better yet, get a group! It's much easier to keep your commitments when you've got others to pull you along. Ask someone to call you on a regular basis to see how you're doing. Choose friends and companions who will support your efforts.

◆ Sign up for a race, a competition, or some other organized event; the exhilaration of completing this will expand your motivation even more. When you've completed one, sign up for the next!

> **Doctors' Orders**
>
> Stop *shoulding* on yourself. Say no to the waiting game and start living life now. Don't wait for the perfect time—there is no perfect time. The right time to start is *now*.

◆ Join a Mastermind Group or some other inspirational organization that will help you to keep your eyes on the prize, or consider hiring a personal coach. The origin of Mastermind Groups (see Appendix B) is attributed to Napoleon Hill, who worked for Andrew Carnegie. The premise is simple: more can be accomplished in less time by working together.

◆ Have a backup plan. The resistance slump is sneaky and bound to hit. When it does, be prepared—who and what will support you to get back on track?

Attention and Commitment

Commit to staying the course for six months. Rome wasn't created in a day, and neither was your current state of health. Give up the defeating notion that you will miraculously change everything in your life in 10 days, as the grocery store checkout line tabloids would have you believe. Consider that you've enrolled yourself in "Clean-Up College" and you're committed to doing whatever it takes to earn your four-year degree.

Loving Yourself at the Start

Appreciate yourself and give yourself healthy rewards along the way. Set up small rewards for small successes and bigger rewards when you've reached your goal. Take care of yourself so you have the energy to pursue your dreams. Be compassionate with yourself and also with the people around you, especially your loved ones— change can be unsettling for many.

Staying Focused on Your Goal

Each week, track your progress and write down your accomplishments. Unless we pay attention, we often lose sight of the fact that we have become what we were seeking. Acknowledge everything you've done and give thanks for what supported you—your inner wisdom, your family, and your friends. *Only then* should you look at what you didn't accomplish. Frame this as, "What was missing this week?" and look to see what you can put in place for success for the following week.

> Mr. Taylor is now cycling to work twice a week and also rides with his sons on weekends. It was hard at first; he felt winded, out of shape, and a little discouraged. With each week he has gradually increased his mileage, and each week he feels stronger. The feeling of exhilaration that he used to get on his bicycle came back to him quickly. If he doesn't feel like exercising, his wife or one of his sons goes out with him to keep him going. He stopped for one week when he got a cold, but his family again helped him to get back on track. He also notices that he is sleeping better and craving less junk food—two added benefits. He is tracking his progress every week. He is clearly in the action phase.

5. Maintenance

Maintenance is the stage for consolidating the gains attained during the action phase and working to prevent relapse. This stage can extend anywhere from six months to indefinitely. In this stage, you start to identify yourself as the person you have become—*I am a healthy man, I am a fitness devotee*, etc. You no longer identify yourself as the one who has failed at attempts at change.

Even with the strongest support systems in place, success ultimately boils down to you. Be proactive. Reassess your goals periodically. If you get off track, you may need a half-time stretch and a revised commitment. This does *not* mean that you throw in the towel!

Watch out for criticism, anger, frustration, self-pity, and other saboteurs. Expect the unexpected and you're on your way to harnessing *everything* for good. Listen to motivational CDs and tapes, watch inspirational movies, and read your favorite success-story books; turn off the television.

6. Termination

The word *termination* was used initially by Dr. Prochaska because it referred to people who were finally terminating substance abuse, such as alcohol or drugs. In this stage, you *know* yourself to be someone different from the person you were in stage 1. You have left the past behind. Your once-new behaviors now feel like a relatively effortless part of your day-to-day rhythm and are easy for you to keep going; they no longer feel like work. Time to take on your next adventure!

> Mr. Taylor returns to his doctor eight months after the previous visit. He has lost 30 pounds, his blood pressure has returned to normal, and he is exercising four times a week. He feels great—he is sleeping well, has plenty of energy, and is savoring the relationships he has with his family. He has organized a cycling team at his company and has been asked to speak at his local community center about how to get in shape in midlife. He is looking ahead to his next goal— a bicycling trip in Italy with his family.

Putting It All Together

Inspiration × Imagination × Commitment × Action = Results! Now that you're ready to make the commitment to change, let's put an action plan into motion. Here's a sample to get you started.

Choose Your Goal

What is calling to you? What makes you light up? What activities cause you to lose your sense of time? Choose a goal for yourself in this realm. (Of course, because you're reading this book, why not start with something that will enhance your health span and your life span? Sometimes the best place to begin is simply with what you love; that in itself will often set the stage for healthy lifestyle behaviors.)

I clearly visualize what my health and my life will look and feel like when I achieve this goal:

_____

_____

Preparation

The steps I will take to prepare for this are ...

_____

_____

Choose Your Action(s)

State a specific action step you will take on a regular basis to achieve your goal. The more specific it is, the more powerful it is. If you don't believe the action is important or if you don't have confidence you can actually do it, then revise your action step until you have something you believe is important and doable. Remember: belief does not always come with thought alone; it comes when thought is combined with action, even in the face of fear, doubt, and resignation.

The action(s) I believe I need to take in order to achieve my goal is (are) ...

_____

_____

Choose Your Support

Create a network of cheerleaders who will support you (translation: hold you accountable!) to do what you said you'd do; for example, an exercise buddy who will rely on you to exercise with her/him.

When I get stuck, the people I can rely on to coach me, support me, and cheer me on are ...

_____

_____

Walt Disney lost millions of dollars and went through multiple setbacks before he finally found success with Mickey Mouse. At one point he was so poor he resorted to eating dog food! Abraham Lincoln was defeated multiple times in many areas of his life before he was elected president in 1860. The lesson here: never give up!

The Least You Need to Know

◆ The six stages for successfully making a change in your life are pre-contemplation, contemplation, preparation, action, maintenance, and termination.

◆ *Intention* is the most powerful beginning to bringing something new into your life.

◆ Clearly imagining your desired and intended outcome will help you stay focused and achieve your goals.

◆ When you find yourself off-course, pay attention to where you got sidelined, line up the support you need to handle it, and get back on track.

◆ Create a structure for action that keeps you focused and on task.

◆ Keep your eyes on the prize, and never give up!

Chapter 21

Spirituality: The Final Frontier

In This Chapter

- ◆ Keeping a positive state of mind
- ◆ The power of spirit
- ◆ Learning grace and gratitude
- ◆ Releasing the past and learning to forgive

When your body is healthy and your mind is vibrant, it's time to focus on your spirit. Spirituality is that dimension of life that lifts us far beyond the limits of our physical bodies. In this final chapter, we'll consider how focusing on your higher consciousness can give your life a sense of peace and meaning. Live the life you were meant to live!

Attitude Is Everything

Modern medicine has taught us that depression, hostility, and loneliness can shorten our life span, perhaps even more than smoking and obesity. However, even those of us who have a tendency toward that "glass half empty" attitude can learn to see the world in a more abundant way; it just takes a little practice and persistence. In the end, longevity is probably best cultivated by creating a positive attitude toward everything in our lives, including our aging bodies, illnesses, and other challenges that we face. Optimism and hope pave the way for new ideas and paths to reveal themselves to us—they take us to places we would never have traveled on our own, revealing exactly what we need for personal growth and healing.

Two people coping with identical illness may have two very different outcomes. One person diagnosed with adult-onset (type 2) diabetes may have constantly elevated blood sugars, progressive organ damage, and may die within 10 years of diagnosis. Another person with the same type of diabetes may have well-controlled blood sugars and live to be 90 or beyond. State of mind is crucial to good outcomes.

To optimize your life span, take a step back and evaluate your relationship with your body and your environment. When you heal your mind and spirit, the positive energy you attain may very well help you increase your longevity. You may find you have the motivation to eat better. You may finally be able to cut down on the drinking. You may be better about taking your daily medications. You may have the energy to seek out new hobbies and new friends.

Tapping Into Spirituality

For some, spirituality may mean religion, but this may not be so for others. Different people seek spirituality from different sources, whether from church or temple, family, volunteering, hobbies, environmental causes, helping those in need, or prayer and meditation.

A sense of spiritual fulfillment will guide you to good health and make caring for your body effortless. How do you utilize spirituality to increase your longevity? You take a break from the 24/7 pace of your life. While you search for the best lab test and the newest prescription to treat your illness, be sure to search for mental peace as well. Cultivate love for yourself, your body, your surroundings, and those around you. Treat yourself with love and kindness, and you will find that your body returns the favor.

Although scientific investigations into the mind-body realm began almost 40 years ago, researchers have only recently begun to explore the beneficial effects of prayer and other spiritual practices on health and healing. There are now over 100 medical schools in the United States that offer courses on spirituality and health, and many of these are part of the required curriculum for medical students.

Renowned cardiologist Herbert Benson at Harvard University is a leader in this field and launched the Harvard conference "Spirituality and Healing in Medicine" in the 1990s. This conference has been held yearly since then, drawing scientists, physicians, theologians, and other seekers from around the world, in a continued attempt to understand how spirit and science interconnect and influence one another. This conference now also addresses the idea that in order to fully understand the influence of consciousness and spirit on the physical body, we may need a whole new way of thinking and of measuring what is possible, of considering that the human body and energy system are greater than the sum of their parts.

> **Words to the Wise**
>
> We shall not cease from exploration, and the end of all our exploring will be to arrive where we started and know the place for the first time.
>
> —T. S. Eliot, poet

Beyond the Physical Plane

A Dartmouth University study published in 1995 looked at the impact of a number of factors on survival in a group of 232 elderly people having elective cardiac surgery. The researchers explored social connections, psychological health, and religious practices. What they found was that those people who either found comfort in their faith or who actively participated in organizations in their community had three times the survival rate compared to those who didn't have these lifelines. Seniors who claimed both of these factors were 10 times as likely to survive.

Why was this happening? We have yet to fully understand how faith, trust, and the will to live impact our survival. The researchers felt, however, that the connection to others, as well as the comfort and trust that faith brought, had a positive impact on survival, perhaps by reducing stress.

Numerous other studies have shown that spiritual beliefs, as well as attendance at a church or other place of worship, offers protection from many diseases, including heart disease, high blood pressure, colitis, and cancer. These effects appear to be independent of one's beliefs or specific spiritual practice and are seen across races, cultures, and continents.

Faith Matters

A 2005 Gallup poll looked at the number of people in the United States who said they believed that God exists. Approximately 78 percent of Americans polled said they were convinced that God indeed exists; 12 percent said they thought this was true but did have some uncertainty. Nine percent were uncertain, and only 1 percent of respondents said they were convinced God does not exist.

Is a religious or spiritual practice important for your health and your longevity? It probably is, especially if you look beyond a traditional definition of God. Considering healing from a spiritual perspective suggests there is a compassionate and loving wisdom and intelligence in the universe (as well as within the individual) available for guidance, support, emotional healing, and even possible physical transformation. As we have already explored in previous chapters, a strong *belief* in something like this often does bring about changes in the physical body.

Larry Dossey, M.D., a physician and leader in the field of alternative medicine, has written extensively about the influence of prayer and intentional focus on numerous biological systems, from yeast and plants to animals and humans. (See Appendix B for one of his books, *Healing Words—The Power of Prayer and the Practice of Medicine*.) While this field is still young, an impressive body of research is accumulating that confirms what many healers have known for centuries: our minds, thoughts, prayers, and intentions do have an impact on our bodies and can influence our environment as well.

Dr. Jeffrey Levin, a renowned social epidemiologist and gerontologist, is a leader in the field of religion, spirituality, and health. One of the first scientists to explore and document the impact of spiritual and religious practices on health outcomes, especially in the elderly, he continues to work on identifying and explaining how prayer and other forms of energy-based medicine help people to heal.

There are several theories as to how spiritual practices might work to help people heal. Spirituality works at different levels:

◆ Many religions expect their followers to adhere to certain health behaviors, such as the avoidance of alcohol, which can have a positive impact on health and increase longevity.

◆ Spiritual practices, such as prayer and meditation, produce relaxation and physiological changes in the body, including the lowering of stress hormones.

◆ Religious organizations provide social interaction and a sense of belonging to a community, which have been shown to improve health and longevity.

Many of these concepts have been ridiculed and considered fringe science by some members of the established medical community, but this view is changing. In fact, views on science in general are undergoing some radical transformations. The field of quantum physics is turning traditional thinking on its ear, and accumulating evidence in this as well as other mind-body disciplines is causing scientists to reevaluate their positions. Many researchers and organizations are now actively exploring the interface of spirituality, medicine, and health and are including them in their studies, including researchers from the National Center for Complementary and Alternative Medicine at the National Institutes of Health.

All-Encompassing Gratitude

The human body is a remarkable, complex machine that performs numerous functions, but it does age. Somewhere along the way your body develops some wear and tear and you develop or contract some diseases along with some serious or not-so-serious medical conditions. You may have to take some medications, and chances are some of your medical problems will cause emotional and physical stress in your life.

Studies have shown that people who experience gratitude tend to be healthier than those who don't feel grateful, and that being grateful changes your perception of life for the better. The health benefits from experiencing gratitude include increased happiness, less depression, the ability to forgive, and the desire to be more helpful.

> **Words to the Wise**
>
> The average man, who does not know what to do with this life, wants another one which shall last forever.
>
> —Anatole France, novelist and literary critic

Clarifying Your Focus

In a 2003 study by P. C. Watkins and colleagues published in the journal *Social Behavior and Personality*, participants were asked to perform a number of different gratitude exercises. These included thinking about a living person for whom they were grateful, writing about a person for whom they were grateful, and writing a letter to deliver to someone for whom they were grateful. Participants who engaged in this experiment showed greater positive emotions afterward. Those who had grateful personalities to begin with showed the greatest benefit from these gratitude exercises.

 Longevity Facts

The longevity secret is not in avoiding all diseases, but in facing them with a healing mind-body approach.

Words to the Wise
Gratitude unlocks the fullness of life. It turns what you have into enough, and more. It turns denial into acceptance, chaos into order, confusion into clarity. It turns problems into gifts, failures into success, the unexpected into perfect timing, and mistakes into important events. Gratitude makes sense of the past, brings peace for today, and creates a vision for tomorrow.   —Melodie Beattie, author

Seeing the Glass Half Full

How you do anything is how you do everything. Your relationship with your body determines the course of your disease. Are you approaching your health from a perspective of anger? If you are suffering from a specific illness, are you resentful of this disease(s)? Are you depressed about your weight? Are you holding on to resentments about personal interactions? Are you avoiding taking responsibility for bad habits such as excessive eating, drinking, or smoking? Are you in a conflicted relationship? If so, then chances are you are not enjoying optimal health.

Focus on what is working in your body—not what is broken. Wake up in gratitude for each new day and with thankfulness for getting this far. Thank your body for what it will be doing for you and promise to care for it. Feel love for your body—the vessel that houses your soul.

Here are some simple ways to practice healing gratitude:

◆ When you wake up, take a few deep breaths before you get out of bed and thank your body for taking care of you while you were sleeping.

◆ As you shower, thank the parts of your body your hands touch.

◆ Look outside and admire the beauty of nature.

◆ Notice the attractiveness of those you love as you encounter them during the day.

◆ Acknowledge people as they help you and make your life easier—from the mail carrier to the grocery clerk.

◆ Be grateful for what is going well in your life.

◆ Notice the parts of your body that work well—these could be your vision, your digestion, or your memory.

◆ Love the parts of your body that don't work well—these could be your heart or your lungs. Notice that these parts are working doubly hard to keep you alive.

Grace and Forgiveness

The eighteenth-century poet, essayist, critic, and satirist Alexander Pope once said, "To err is human, to forgive, divine." Forgiving, however, is hard to do. Most of us have anger or hurt about various events that have happened to us. We may be holding on to these feelings, unable to let go. We may focus more on the negativity of these events than we do on what is good in our lives.

Here's a story to illustrate what can happen when we aren't willing to let go. An ancient technique in India for catching a monkey was to carve a hole in a coconut and place a banana inside. The hole was big enough for a monkey's paw to slip inside, but not big enough for the monkey to withdraw his closed fist holding the banana. The hunters then attached the coconut to a tree and waited for a monkey to come along and grab the banana. Once the monkey's paw was inside the coconut, capture was usually inevitable because of the monkey's unwillingness to drop the banana, even though letting go would allow the monkey to escape.

Releasing the Past

Just like the monkey and the coconut, we hold on to negative thoughts even though we know they are causing us pain, depression, and hurt. Letting go of these thoughts and focusing on the good in our lives makes us emotionally healthier, and that often leads to better physical health as well.

Dr. Fred Luskin, founder of the Stanford University Forgiveness Project, has done pioneering research on the impact of forgiveness on both mental and physical health. His studies have shown that forgiveness training leads to improvements in the cardiovascular and nervous systems, as well as relaxation and improved emotions. Conversely, he has also shown that when people actively hold and nurse their grudges, their blood pressure, heart rate, muscle tension, and arterial wall stress increase. Both forgiveness and grudge-holding are states of mind that produce immediate emotional and physical responses in the body.

Other studies have shown that the more forgiving people become, the fewer physical symptoms and illnesses they experience. Most of the studies done to date are short term, and while there is not yet a lot of data on the impact of forgiveness on survival and longevity, this relationship may become more clearly defined in the near future.

Determining Hurt

How do you know if a past hurt or event is causing you significant stress in your life? See if you answer yes to the following questions:

◆ Does the memory of a past event arouse strong negative emotions in you— emotions such as anger, resentment, frustration, hurt, or a sense of unfairness or hopelessness?

◆ Do you find yourself unable to turn off angry or painful thoughts once you start having them?

◆ Do you find yourself going through the same thought processes over and over again?

◆ Do you find your negative feelings or thoughts about an event intruding on your daily activities and relationships?

If you've answered yes to any these questions, chances are you are holding on to something you need to forgive. That persistent perception of hurt may harm your health span and may even negatively impact your life span. Common areas that present the opportunity to forgive can include pain around abusive or dysfunctional relationships in childhood, conflicted romantic relationships, work issues, divorce, and physical or sexual abuse.

How does one forgive? By choosing to let go of the hurt and allowing peace to take its place. You don't have to absolve the wrongdoer of guilt or responsibility, nor do you have to forgive the crime itself. You just have to make a decision not to allow past events with negative emotions to take up present space in your head. Sometimes forgiveness comes more readily when you can identify something that you learned from the event, perhaps some way in which it made you stronger, wiser, or more compassionate. This takes practice and persistence; sometimes you may need to forgive many times before you finally feel at peace. You may find, at times, that forgiving is difficult. At these times, seeking help through counseling can guide you through that process. You may also find solace in spiritual counseling, journaling, meditation, or self-help groups.

Doctors' Orders

People who forgive report fewer health problems, have fewer physical symptoms of stress, and feel better psychologically and emotionally. People who hold on to blame and anger have a higher incidence of cardiovascular disease, high blood pressure, cancer, muscle tension, and a depressed immune response.

There is a saying that "Resentment is a poison you keep taking, hoping for the other person to die." The negative emotions that you harbor and keep reliving certainly can be poisonous to your health. Find ways to let them go and lead a longer, happier life.

Creating Your Own Life Story

You, and only you, have a chance to write your life story. Will you cast yourself as the hero or heroine, living one vibrant adventure after another? Will you be someone well-loved who spread love abundantly? Will you be a person who led a rich and fulfilled life, took chances, and had no regrets? If so, then you are on the right track.

That same life lived could have been, instead, the story of a victim, of hurts suffered, pain borne, missed chances, failed attempts, and misery.

How are you going to view your life? What role will you nurture and expand? It's up to you. Pick and choose what you want to remember and paint it any color of emotion you want. For an emotionally healthy life span, choose to let go of the hurts that hold you back and look back in gratitude and wonder at the life and body that have brought you this far.

Creating Your Future

Cancer survivors often have a unique view on life—they have been given the gift of enjoying each day and the miracles that it brings. What if we all chose to do the same with our lives? Most of us live life putting away our happiness until we have all our ducks in a row. That day may never come. Most of us think we will live to 90. What if you don't? You have but one life to live, so envision a vibrant future filled with possibilities, health, and happiness. By enjoying the present moment—the here and now—you are making the most of your short time on Earth, whatever your longevity karma may be.

Giving Back

Volunteering is good for you! As you saw in Chapter 9, altruism is good for both the giver and the receiver. Philanthropy of either time or money can be extremely spiritually satisfying.

In a 1988 study of more than 3,000 volunteers, Allen Luks surveyed the relationship between helping and good health. Survey respondents noticed a "helpers high"—a rush of euphoria that was related to the act of volunteering. Approximately 57 percent of the volunteers mentioned an increased sense of self-worth, and 53 percent noted such gains as greater happiness and optimism, as well as a decrease in feelings of helplessness and depression. Many other studies have reproduced what this survey discovered.

Goodness of Heart and Greatness of Being

What is good is great, and greatness can be achieved in the peace of your garden, in the twinkle of your grandchild's eyes, and in the wisdom of acceptance of life's challenges. Greatness can be in the courageous recovery from disease or a traumatic life event. It can be the courage to heal and the ability to let go of pain. It can be in the acceptance of loss and the strength to keep on going. It can be found in prayer and meditation. It can be seen in facing loneliness and in the creation of a new life for oneself.

Goodness and greatness in your health arise from ignoring the pessimistic, avoiding the petty, and stepping away from the negative. Instead, with greatness, you focus on what is right and keep an optimistic attitude toward your health. This will strengthen your personal longevity and carry you through life's roller-coaster ride.

The Secret to Longevity Is Your Personality

What personality characteristics are associated with a long life? Findings from the 2006 Tokyo Centenarian Study suggest that high scores in the specific personality traits of conscientiousness, extraversion, and openness are associated with increased longevity. Why? It is thought that these personality traits contribute to longevity through health-related behavior, stress reduction, and adaptation to the challenges we face as we get older.

Knowing that your personality can impact your life span, how do you create your longevity personality? *Character Strengths and Virtues* by Christopher Peterson and Martin Seligman (Oxford University Press, 2004) identifies six classes of virtues. These positive psychological traits are well worth cultivating, and include:

1. *Wisdom and knowledge:* Creativity, curiosity, open-mindedness, love of learning, perspective

2. *Courage:* Bravery, persistence, integrity, vitality

3. *Humanity:* Love, kindness, social intelligence

4. *Justice:* Citizenship, fairness, leadership

5. *Temperance:* Forgiveness and mercy, humility and modesty, prudence, self-regulation

6. *Transcendence:* Appreciation of beauty and excellence, gratitude, hope, humor, spirituality

As you've perused the pages of this book, you have heard from doctors and medical experts, but what about the true longevity experts—the ones who have walked the walk? What they have to offer is well worth considering. Olive Watson is a vibrant, energetic, and articulate 100-year-old former nurse who enjoys excellent health. When asked about her personal secrets of longevity, she offered the following thoughts:

◆ Eat right; eat of the earth. Eat food in its most natural state.

◆ Find spiritual fulfillment. This will become your reason for living.

◆ Stay active, and accept that your body will age. You will need to keep changing your activities to fit your body's capacities.

◆ Moderate your activities with age—you will find that you need to do them at a less rushed pace, with more rests in between.

◆ Age with grace, and keep your mind and body going!

Good footsteps to follow! You can create your own destiny and decide how you will live this wonderful life. Perhaps this longevity affirmation will inspire you to create one of your own: "I choose to create a future for myself that is healthy and happy. I will be grateful to my body for the work it does and treat it well by feeding and exercising it properly, by resting it when it is tired, and by giving it healing when it becomes ill. I will fulfill my soul by honoring its desires, and will fulfill my destiny by courageously stepping into the path I am meant to follow. And, when it is over, I will have lived a good life."

The Least You Need to Know

◆ Positive personality traits have been shown to have lasting health benefits.

◆ Forgiveness of past hurts is important to future health.

◆ You may not be able to change your life events, but your perception of those events changes your health.

◆ Gratitude, goodness of heart, and a sense of spiritual fulfillment are positive traits associated with good health.

◆ The true longevity secret may lie not only in a long life, but a life well-lived and full of meaning.

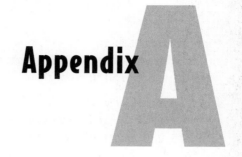

Glossary

acid reflux disease   *See* GERD (gastroesophageal reflux disease).

aerobic exercise   Often referred to as endurance exercise. Exercise that makes your heart rate increase, gets your blood pumping, and makes you breathe harder.

aneurysm   Bulge in a blood vessel; dangerous, because it may burst.

antioxidants   Nutrients or chemicals such as vitamin C that quench or neutralize free radicals and prevent them from causing damage.

arthritis   Refers to inflammation of the joints and is a grab-bag term that includes over 100 different types of conditions, including gout, osteoarthritis, autoimmune arthritis such as rheumatoid arthritis, and fibromyalgia.

atherosclerosis   *See* coronary artery disease.

audiometric evaluation   Series of tests, conducted by a licensed clinical audiologist, to discover how well you hear, as well as to detect any conditions or abnormalities that may affect your hearing or your balance.

autophagy   Ability of a cell to literally devour and remove parts of itself that are old and unhealthy and that, left untouched, could harm the cell.

bariatric surgery   Refers to medical operations designed to promote weight loss. *See also* gastric banding, gastric bypass, and vertical banded gastroplasty.

barium enema   Material used to highlight structures during X-rays of the lower gastrointestinal tract.

bio-identical hormones   Hormone products chemically identical to those made in human ovaries; they include estradiol, estrone, estriol, progesterone, and testosterone. All of these natural hormones are actually made in a laboratory.

biogerontology   Field of geriatrics dedicated to the study of the biological changes associated with aging. Some researchers in this field, known as biomedical gerontologists, also hope to discover ways to extend life and prevent or even reverse aging. They feel humans are probably capable of living to 150 or longer, given the right circumstances.

biological age   An estimate of age based on one's health parameters, using biomarkers such as blood pressure, muscle strength, and blood sugar level.

biomarker   Physical characteristic or trait indicative of one's biological age or risk of illness.

body dysmorphic disorder   Condition in which individuals have a distorted or exaggerated view of their appearance and become obsessed with their physical characteristics or perceived flaws.

body lift   Surgical procedure that removes excess fat and skin and improves the appearance of cellulite or dimpling in the skin.

carotid ultrasound   Test using Doppler ultrasound to get a picture of the arteries leading to the brain.

catechins   Powerful antioxidants felt to exert cancer protective benefits. Green tea probably has the highest amount, followed by oolong and then black tea.

chemical peel   Chemical solution applied to the skin to burn off the outer layers. The skin that appears is smoother with fewer fine wrinkles and fewer pigmentation changes.

cholesterol   Fatty, waxy substance produced naturally in the liver. Cholesterol levels refer to a group of lipids or fats in the bloodstream—the result of how much the liver makes, along with what your diet contributes. Total cholesterol is the total amount of cholesterol measured in your blood; a normal level is now considered under 200. *See also* HDL cholesterol and LDL cholesterol.

chronological age   The number of years a person has actually lived.

clitoral suction device   Device that pulls the blood supply to the surface of the clitoris to enhance sensation and orgasm during sex.

colonoscopy Procedure to look inside the rectum and colon for polyps, abnormal areas, or cancer.

core muscles Muscles of the trunk, from the shoulders and spine down to the hips, that provide stability and help to maintain good posture.

coronary artery disease Also known as atherosclerosis, refers to blockage in the arteries that supply blood to the heart muscle.

dermatology Branch of medicine dealing with the skin and its appendages (hair, nails, and sweat glands). A dermatologist is a medical doctor who specializes in this area.

DHEA (dehydroepiandrosterone) Steroid hormone produced by the adrenal glands. It acts on the body much like testosterone and is converted into testosterone and estrogen.

diabetes Common term for the medical condition known as diabetes mellitus, in which the body's blood sugar is higher than normal.

digital rectal exam (DRE) Generally part of the yearly physical exam. The doctor or nurse inserts a lubricated, gloved finger into the lower part of the rectum to feel for lumps or anything else that seems unusual.

DNA-based tests *See* gene tests.

EKG treadmill test Test in which a patient walks on a treadmill at increasing speeds, while hooked up to an EKG; changes in the tracing of the EKG during exercise are used to assess the possibility of heart disease.

electrolysis Traditional semipermanent method that cauterizes and destroys each individual hair follicle.

endorphins Morphinelike chemicals produced in the brain that reduce pain and produce a sense of well-being. They are nature's own painkillers.

epigenetics Science that looks at how certain environmental factors, particularly certain chemicals and nutrients, may have an impact on how our genes are switched on and off.

erectile dysfunction (ED) The inability to achieve or maintain an erection.

free radicals Molecules with an unstable unpaired electron capable of damaging other molecules or cells. Free radicals are generated by normal metabolism in cells, as well as by things in the environment such as cigarette smoke and radiation.

gastric banding   A procedure that involves placing a silicone band around the upper part of the stomach and tightening it to create a small upper stomach through which food must pass.

gastric bypass   A procedure most commonly done is called the Roux-en-Y procedure. This operation reduces the stomach to a small pouch. Part of the small intestine is then bypassed, and the remaining small intestine is attached to the stomach pouch. Patients lose up to 80 percent of their excess weight with this type of procedure.

gene tests   Also called DNA-based tests, laboratory tests for genetic disorders an individual may have. Involve direct examination of the DNA molecule itself. The DNA sample can be obtained from any tissue, including blood.

genetic testing   The process of analyzing someone's genetic material, or DNA, to look for specific changes in genes that might indicate an increased risk of certain disease, including cancer. Genetic screening is usually done with a simple blood test.

genetics   The science of heredity and variation in human beings. It is based on the premise that molecules called DNA make up the genetic code of an individual and patterns in this genetic code determine various traits and states of a disease.

GERD (gastroesophageal reflux disease)   Acid reflux disease. GERD occurs when the lower esophageal sphincter doesn't close properly and allows acid to back up into the esophagus.

gerontology   The study of the biological, psychological, and sociological aspects connected with the aging process. A *gerontologist* is a physician specializing in these areas.

glycemic index   Refers to how quickly a particular food, especially a carb, is absorbed and converted into sugar in the blood stream.

HDL cholesterol   Good cholesterol. Men should have a level over 40, and women should be over 50.

health span   The percentage of your life span that is spent in good health, where you have the energy and the vitality to pursue the activities important to you.

homocysteine   Amino acid produced in the body, usually as a by-product of consuming meat.

hormones   Chemical substances produced in the body that control and regulate the activity of certain cells or organs.

hydrogenated fat *See* trans fat.

IgA One of several types of antibodies produced by some of our white blood cells. It is found mainly in body fluids, including saliva and tears, where it helps to fight off bacteria, viruses, and other unwelcome visitors.

immunizations Injections given to trigger the immune system to be able to recognize and attack future disease. If you are exposed to the full-blown disease later in life, you will either not become infected or have a much less serious infection.

immunosuppression Term used for the inhibition of the normal functioning of our infection-fighting white blood cells.

insomnia Difficulty falling asleep or staying asleep, or the inability to achieve restful sleep.

insulin Hormone made by the pancreas. It is considered one of the master regulators of metabolism in the body and is primarily responsible for the metabolism of glucose. If insulin becomes deficient or if it stops working efficiently, then diabetes develops.

kegels Named for Dr. Arnold Kegel, these are exercises designed to strengthen the muscles that stop urination. These muscles are also used during sexual intercourse.

LDL cholesterol Bad cholesterol. A good LDL is under 130; an optimal level is under 100.

legumes The fruits or seeds of plants such as beans, peas, and lentils.

life span The maximum time an organism can be expected to survive. In humans, this is generally around 120 years.

lymphatic system A major component of the immune system that helps remove excess fluids from body tissues. The lymphatic system is a network of lymphoid organs, lymph nodes, lymph ducts, lymphatic tissues, lymph capillaries, and lymph vessels that produce and transport lymph fluid from tissues to the circulatory system.

mammography Low-dose x-ray used to examine the breasts to aid in the diagnosis of breast diseases in women.

manopause (andropause) The reduction in the production of certain chemicals such as testosterone and DHEA by the body, and the health effects associated with the decreased levels of these chemicals.

massage therapy   Term used to define a process in which therapists press, rub, and manipulate muscles and soft tissues with pressure from their hands or other parts of their body. Massage is used to decrease pain and relax the soft tissues and muscles, with the typical massage session lasting anywhere from 30 minutes to 1 hour.

mcgm   Abbreviation for microgram.

meditation   Ancient practice of stilling the incessant activity of the mind, usually by focusing on breathing, an object, or a word.

menopause   The cessation ("pause") of the menstrual cycle for one year or more. Average age in the United States is 51 years (the range is 40–58 years).

metabolic syndrome   Also known as Syndrome X, a cluster of risk factors that, in combination, greatly increase the risk of diabetes and cardiovascular disease.

metastasis   Name given to the process of distant spread of malignant tumors.

mg   Abbreviation for milligram.

microdermabrasion   Process in which the dead outer surface (stratum corneum) of the skin is removed. This is done with mechanical abrasion through a handheld wand, using particles such as zinc oxide or aluminum oxide crystals that rub against the skin. Microdermabrasion also stimulates the production of skin cells and collagen.

minerals   Essential components of blood, organs, and other tissues. Minerals also drive the body's enzyme systems, allowing biochemical reactions to take place.

morbidity   Pattern of disease or illness seen in a population.

MRA (Magnetic Resonance Angiography)   Combines the MRI with contrast material to get a picture of the arteries. This can provide further information about the vessels leading to the brain and those in the brain and can reveal aneurisms, blockages, and dissections in the brain vessels.

MRI (Magnetic Resonance Imaging)   Uses a magnetic field to get pictures of soft tissues and bones inside the body. It is the most sensitive test to get a picture of the brain. Used to help diagnose brain tumors, aneurysms, strokes, signs of trauma, and other disorders of the nervous system, such as vasculitis and multiple sclerosis.

nanotechnology   The engineering of functional systems at the molecular level.

natural hormones   *See* bio-identical hormones.

neuropathy   Loosely translates into pain in the nerve endings. Peripheral neuropathy can be a caused by longstanding uncontrolled diabetes but may also be caused by chronic alcoholism, nutritional deficiencies, or certain infections.

neurotransmitter   Chemical messenger released by a cell that travels to a nearby or distant cell to relay information. Once thought to only be produced by neurons (cells of the nervous system), neurotransmitters have been found to be produced and also received by nearly every tissue in the body.

osteoarthritis   Refers to wear and tear of the joints.

osteoporosis   Refers to thinning of the bones.

pap smear   Sample of cells from the cervix to check for early changes suggestive of cervical cancer.

parabens   Preservative used in deodorants and antiperspirants, acts like an estrogen in the body.

pedometer   Small device usually worn at the waist that measures how many steps you take each day.

penile implants   Surgically placed inside the penis for men suffering from complete impotence. An implanted pump in the groin or scrotum is manipulated by hand—this pump is attached to a reservoir and fills cylinders placed in the penis to achieve an erection. The erection can be controlled in terms of duration, amount, and timing.

penile pump   Cylindrical device placed over the penis, with a manual or motorized pump to create suction. As the apparatus creates a vacuum around the penis, blood is drawn into the penis, helping it to become engorged. This mechanical suction helps to achieve an erection.

peripheral artery disease (PAD)   Condition similar to coronary artery disease. In PAD, fatty deposits build up in the inner linings of the artery walls, restricting blood circulation. This can occur in arteries leading to the kidneys, stomach, arms, legs, and feet.

phthalates   Chemicals used to make plastic products softer and more pliable.

phytochemicals   Chemicals present in a plant considered to have a beneficial effect on human health. These include polyphenols, indoles, organosulfides, terpines, and organic acids. *See also* polyphenols.

plaque   Formed from cholesterol, fat, calcium, and other substances in the blood. When blood cholesterol levels are high, there is a greater chance that plaque will build up on the artery walls.

polyphenols   Chemical substances found in plants that contain a phenol group, such as tanins, lignins, and flavanoids. Sources of polyphenols include berries, tea, grapes, walnuts, and pomegranates. *See also* phytochemicals.

positive self-talk   Practice of replacing negative, self-critical thinking with positive, productive affirmations.

psychoneuroimmunology   Emerging science exploring the mind's intricate relation to the workings of the body and vice versa.

resveratrol   Plant nutrient found in red wine and the skin of red grapes. Resveratrol has anti-inflammatory actions, protects many tissues in the body (including the heart), and also seems to protect against cancer.

senescence   Biological changes associated with an aging body.

sigmoidoscopy   Procedure that looks inside the rectum and lower (sigmoid) colon for polyps, abnormal areas, or cancer.

SPF (sun protection factor)   In a sunscreen, indicates the length of time a person can be exposed to sunlight before getting sunburn with protection compared to how long the skin takes to redden without protection.

statins   Cholesterol-lowering medications that also stabilize plaque in arteries.

stress   Condition of mental, emotional, or physical upset or strain that generally produces chemical and physical changes in the body, including an outpouring of adrenaline, increased muscle tension, and elevated heart rate and blood pressure.

stress echocardiogram   Similar to a stress EKG, except that an echocardiogram picture of your heart is also obtained, both at rest and during exercise.

strokes   "Brain attacks" that occur when blood clots form in blood vessels that supply the brain. The blood vessels narrow as a result of these clots, and the blood supply to the brain is cut off. Bleeding within the brain can occur and brain damage and death may result.

successful aging   Aging that is unaccompanied by chronic disease and disability.

supplements   Vitamins, minerals, herbs and spices, other botanicals or plant chemicals, and mixtures of these categories, such as multivitamin/mineral pills.

Syndrome X   *See* metabolic syndrome.

trans fat (hydrogenated fat)   A polyunsaturated oil (such as corn oil) that has been turned into a solid fat (such as margarine or vegetable shortening) by exposing it to high heat and pressure.

tumor   An overgrowth of cells in the body. A *benign tumor* does not spread to tissues around it or to distant parts of the body; it is not necessarily life threatening. A *malignant tumor* is a life-threatening, cancerous growth that invades tissues and disrupts the function of the healthy organs around it; can spread to other parts of the body.

UVAs   Longwave solar rays less likely to cause sunburn but can enhance UVBs' cancer-causing effects. UVA rays penetrate more deeply and are a chief cause of wrinkling and leathering of the skin. UV refers to ultraviolet. A and B are types of ultraviolet rays.

UVBs   Shortwave solar rays extremely potent in producing sunburn. Exposure to these rays causes three different types of skin cancer: basal cell, squamous cell, and melanoma.

vertical banded gastroplasty   Operation in which the stomach is simply reduced to a pouch that severely restricts the amount of food one can eat before feeling full. The small intestine is not involved.

vitamins   Natural compounds found in plant and animal food; needed in relatively small quantities but are essential for life.

Resources

If you want to learn more, start with these books, websites, and other resources, organized by chapter topic.

Chapter 1: Seeking a Great Health Span

Chopra, Deepak, M.D., and David Simon, M.D. *Grow Younger, Live Longer.* New York: Three Rivers Press, 2001.

Roizen, Michael D., M.D. *The Real Age Makeover.* New York: Collins/ HarperCollins, 2004.

Rowe, John W., M.D., and Robert Kahn, Ph.D. *Successful Aging.* New York: Dell Publishing, 1998.

Weil, Andrew, M.D. *Healthy Aging—A Lifelong Guide to Your Well-Being.* New York: Random House, 2005.

Wilcox, Bradley J., D. Craig Wilcox, and Makoto Suzuki. *The Okinawa Program: How the World's Longest-Lived People Achieve Everlasting Health—And How You Can Too.* New York: Clarkson Potter, 2001.

Living to 100: Life Expectancy Calculator—Thomas Perls, M.D., M.Ph., The New England Centenarian Study www.livingto100.com

National Institute on Aging—www.nia.nih.gov

Chapter 2: Understanding Your Longevity Group

Centers for Disease Control (CDC)—"About Minority Health," www.cdc.gov/omhd/ AMA/AMH.htm

Centers for Disease Control (CDC)—"Fact Sheet CDC Division of Media Relations: Racial Ethnic Health Disparities," www.cdc.gov/od/oc/medica/pressrel/ fs040402.htm

National Cancer Institute—"Elements of Cancer Genetics Risk Assessment and Counseling," www.cancer.gov/cancertopics/pdq/genetics/ risk-assessment-and-counseling

Scientific and Educational Website on Human Longevity—"Genetics: Ethnicity. MacMillan Encyclopedia of Aging," www.longevity-science.org/ Genetics-Ethnicity.htm

Chapter 3: Keeping Healthy, Keeping Track

Evans, William, Ph.D., and Irwin H. Rosenberg, M.D., with Jacqueline Thompson. *Biomarkers: The 10 Keys to Prolonging Vitality*. New York: Simon & Schuster, 1991.

Hankinson, Susan, R.N., Sc.D., Graham A. Colditz, M.D., Dr.PH., JoAnn E. Manson, M.D., Dr.PH., and Frank E. Speizer, M.D., eds. *Healthy Women, Healthy Lives—A Guide to Preventing Disease, from the Landmark Nurses' Health Study*. New York: Simon & Schuster, 2001.

National Society of Genetic Counselors (NSGC)—"Your Family History—Your Future," www.nsgc.org/consumer/familytree

U.S. Department of Health and Human Services, Healthy People 2010—"Leading Health Indicators," www.healthypeople.gov/Document/HTML/uih/uih_4.htm

U.S. Preventive Services Task Force (USPSTF) Guide to Clinical Preventive Services, 2006, www.ahrq.gov/clinic/pocketgd/.htm

Chapter 4: Nutrition for Life

Bauer, Joy, M.S., R.D., C.D.N. *The Complete Idiot's Guide to Total Nutrition*. Indianapolis: Alpha Books, 2005.

Campbell, T. Colin, Ph.D., and Thomas M. Campbell II. *The China Study.* Dallas: Benbella Books, 2006.

Heber, David, M.D., Ph.D., with Susan Bowerman, M.S., R.D. *What Color Is Your Diet?* New York: Regan Books/Harper Collins, 2001.

Walford, Roy L., and Lisa Walford. *The Anti-Aging Plan: The Nutrient-Rich, Low-Calorie Way of Eating for a Longer Life—The Only Diet Scientifically Proven to Extend Your Healthy Years.* New York: Marlowe & Company, 2005.

Weil, Andrew, M.D. *Eating Well for Optimum Health.* New York: HarperCollins, 2001.

Willett, Walter, M.D., Dr.PH. *Eat, Drink and Be Healthy—The Harvard Medical School Guide to Healthy Eating.* New York: Free Press/Simon & Schuster, 2001.

Center for Science in the Public Interest—Nutrition Action Health Letter, www.cspinet.org

Timothy S. Harlan, M.D.—The gourmet healthy chef who's also an Internal Medicine doctor, http://drgourmet.com

Tufts University Health & Nutrition Letter, http://healthletter.tufts.edu

USDA Food Pyramid, http://www.mypyramid.gov

Chapter 5: Exercise Essentials

Moffat, Marilyn, P.T., Ph.D., and Carole B. Lewis, P.T., Ph.D. *Age Defying Fitness: Making the Most of Your Body for the Rest of Your Life.* Atlanta: Peachtree Publishers, 2006.

Nelson, Miriam E., Ph.D., with Sarah Wernick, Ph.D. *Strong Women Stay Young.* New York: Bantam Books, 1998.

The Yoga Journal and Timothy McCall, M.D. *Yoga as Medicine: The Yogic Prescription for Health and Healing.* New York: Bantam, 2007.

American College of Sports Medicine, www.acsm.org/AM/Template.cfm?Section=Home

American Council on Exercise, www.acefitness.org

Centers for Disease Control and Prevention—Physical Activity Topics—great resource, www.cdc.gov/nccdphp/dnpa/physical/index.htm

Dept of Health and Human Services—Info on how to get fit, healthy diets, etc.; has an online activity tracker, www.smallstep.gov

Exercise: A Guide from the National Institutes on Aging, www.nia.nih.gov/exercisebook

Chapter 6: Ousting Obesity, Increasing Longevity

Carson, Carole. *From Fat to Fit*. Nevada City, CA: Hound Press, 2007.

Fletcher, Anne M., M.S., R.D. *Thin for Life: 10 Keys to Success from People Who Have Lost Weight and Kept It Off*. New York: Houghton Mifflin, 2003.

Katzen, Mollie, and Walter Willett, M.D. *Eat, Drink, and Weigh Less*. New York: Hyperion, 2007.

Rolls, Barbara, Ph.D. *Volumetrics Weight Control Plan*. New York: HarperCollins, 2000.

Shapiro, Howard M., M.D. *Dr. Shapiro's Picture Perfect Weight Loss*. New York: Rodale, 2000.

National Weight Control Registry, www.nwcr.ws

Chapter 7: Supplements

Many of the books listed in Chapter 4 on nutrition offer valuable resources on supplements.

American Botanical Council, http://abc.herbalgram.org/site/PageServer

Consumer Lab—An independent testing lab offering information on the purity of numerous supplements; also has a great database of information about supplements. Costs about $30 per year, www.consumerlab.com

National Center for Complementary and Alternative Medicine, NIH, http://nccam.nih.gov

National Institutes of Health, Office of Dietary Supplements, http://dietary-supplements.info.nih.gov

United States FDA, Center for Food Safety and Applied Nutrition, Dietary Supplements, www.cfsan.fda.gov/~dms/supplmnt.html

Chapter 8: Creating Restorative Sleep

Dement, William C., M.D., Ph.D., and Christopher Vaughan. *The Promise of Sleep: A Pioneer in Sleep Medicine Explores the Vital Connection Between Health, Happiness, and a Good Night's Sleep.* New York: Bantam Dell, 2000.

Epstein, Lawrence, M.D., with Steven Mardon. *The Harvard Medical School Guide to a Good Night's Sleep.* New York: McGraw-Hill, 2006.

American Academy of Sleep Medicine, www.aasmnet.org

American Insomnia Association, www.americaninsomniaassociation.org/home.asp

National Sleep Foundation, www.sleepfoundation.org/site/c.huIXKjM0IxF/b.2417141/k.2E30/The_National_Sleep_Foundation.htm

Chapter 9: Touch, Connection, and Sex

Butler, Robert N., M.D., and Myrna Lewis, A.C.S.W. *Love and Sex After 40: A Guide for Men and Women for Their Mid and Later Years.* New York: HarperCollins, 1986.

Deida, David. *Intimate Communion: Awakening Your Sexual Essence.* Deerfield Beach, FL: Health Communications, Inc., 1995.

Holstein, Lana, M.D. *How to Have Magnificent Sex.* New York: Random House, 2003.

Love, Pat, Ed.D. *Hot Monogamy.* New York: Penguin Group, 1995.

Schnarch, David, Ph.D. *Passionate Marriage: Love, Sex and Intimacy in Emotionally Committed Relationships.* New York: W.W. Norton & Company, 1997.

MayoClinic.com—"Massage: A relaxing method to relieve stress and pain," www.mayoclinic.com/health/massage/SA00082

National Center for Complementary and Alternative Medicine—"Massage Therapy as CAM," www.nccam.nih.gov/health/massage

Chapter 10: Your Healthy Heart

Arnot, Bob, M.D. *Seven Steps to Stop a Heart Attack.* New York: Simon & Schuster, 2005.

Ornish, Dean, M.D. *Dr. Dean Ornish's Program for Reversing Heart Disease.* New York: Ballantine Books, 1990.

——— *Love and Survival.* New York: Harper Collins, 1998.

Superko, H. Robert, M.D., with Laura Tucker. *Before the Heart Attacks: A Revolutionary Approach to Detecting, Preventing, and Even Reversing Heart Disease.* New York: Rodale, 2003.

The American Heart Association, www.americanheart.org

The American Heart Association—A free physical activity program for women to help incorporate fitness into your life, www.choosetomove.org

National Heart, Lung, and Blood Institute, National Institutes of Health, www.nhlbi. nih.gov/index.htm

U.S. Department of Health and Human Services, Women's Heart Health, www. womenshealth.gov/hearttruth/index.cfm

Chapter 11: Getting the Fighting Edge on Cancer

Gaynor, Mitchell L., M.D. *Nurture Nature Nurture Health: Your Health and the Environment.* New York: Nurture Nature Press, 2005.

Hirshberg, Caryle, and Marc Ian Barasch. *Remarkable Recovery.* New York: Riverhead Books, 1995.

LeShan, Lawrence, Ph.D. *Cancer as a Turning Point.* New York: Plume/Penguin, 1989.

Siegel, Bernie, M.D. *Love, Medicine, and Miracles.* New York: HarperCollins, 1986.

Simonton, O. Carl, M.D., James L. Creighton, Ph.D., and Stephanie Matthews. *Getting Well Again.* New York: Bantam, 1992.

Spiegel, David, M.D. *Living Beyond Limits.* New York: Ballantine Books, 1993.

American Cancer Society, www.cancer.org/docroot/home/index.asp

Centers for Disease Control (CDC), www.cdc.gov/cancer/

Environmental Working Group, www.ewg.org/featured/169

Gaynor Integrative Oncology—Mitchell Gaynor, M.D., www.gaynoroncology. com/gaynor/new/en/default/view/3/

"Meditations for Enhancing Your Immune System," audio CD by Bernie Siegel, M.D., Hay House, 1998.

National Cancer Institute, www.cancer.gov

Chapter 12: Vital Lungs

Centers for Disease Control—"Health Effects of Cigarette Smoking," www.cdc.gov/tobacco/data_statistics/Factsheets/health_effects.htm

National Heart, Lung, and Blood Institute—"It has a name: COPD (Chronic Obstructive Pulmonary Disease," www.LearnAboutCOPD.org

Chapter 13: Keeping Your Brain Healthy

Bierman, Judy, and Barbara Toohey. *The Stroke Book*. New York: Penguin, 2005.

Khalsa, Dharma Singh, M.D., with Cameron Stauth. *Brain Longevity*. New York: Warner Books, 1997.

Perlmutter, David, M.D., and Carol Colman. *The Better Brain Book*. New York: Penguin Group, 2004.

Victoroff, Jeff, M.D. *Saving Your Brain: The Revolutionary Plan to Boost Brain Power, Improve Memory, and Protect Yourself Against Aging and Alzheimer's.* New York: Bantam Books, 2003.

AARP—"Aging Successfully, and Myths About Aging and the Brain," www.aarp.org/health/brain/aging/myths_about_aging_and_the_brain.html

Chapter 14: Say No to Diabetes

American Diabetes Association, www.diabetes.org

American Diabetes Association—"How to Prevent Pre-Diabetes," www.diabetes.org/pre-diabetes/what-you-can-do.jsp

American Diabetes Association—"Your Body's Well Being," www.diabetes.org/type-2-diabetes/well-being.jsp

National Diabetes Information Clearing House—"Diabetes Overview," www.diabetes.niddk.nih.gov/dm/pubs/overview/index.htm

Chapter 15: Musculoskeletal Health

Sarno, John, M.D. *Healing Back Pain.* New York: Warner Books, 1991.

Vickery, Steve, and Marilyn Moffat, P.T., Ph.D. *The American Physical Therapy Association Book of Body Maintenance and Repair.* New York: Holt Paperbacks, 1999.

The Arthritis Foundation, www.arthritis.org

National Institute of Arthritis and Musculoskeletal and Skin Diseases (NIAMS)—www.niams.nih.gov; toll-free in the U.S.: 1-877-22-NIAMS

National Osteoporosis Foundation (NOF)—www.NOF.org; 1232 22nd Street N.W., Washington, D.C. 20037-1202; 800-231-4222; 202-223-2226

Chapter 16: Hormones and Longevity

Kagan, Leslee, M.S., N.P., Bruce Kessel, M.D., and Herbert Benson, M.D. *Mind Over Menopause: The Complete Mind/Body Approach to Coping with Menopause.* New York: Free Press/Simon & Schuster, 2004.

Love, Susan M., M.D., with Karen Lindsey. *Dr. Susan Love's Hormone Book.* New York: Times Books/Random House, 1998.

Northrup, Christiane, M.D. *The Wisdom of Menopause.* New York: Bantam, 2006.

Pelletier, Maureen Miller, M.D., and Deborah S. Romaine. *The Complete Idiot's Guide to Menopause.* Indianapolis: Alpha Books, 2000.

North American Menopause Society, www.menopause.org/default.htm

Chapter 17: Look Younger, Feel Younger

The American Academy of Dermatology, www.aad.org

The American Dermatological Association, www.amer-derm-assn.org

American Society of Plastic Surgeons, www.plasticsurgery.org

WebMD—"Cosmetic Surgery Self Assessment," www.webmd.com/content/pages/14/89109.htm

Chapter 18: Unlocking the Power and Potential of Your Mind

Begley, Sharon. *Train Your Mind, Change Your Brain*. New York: Ballantine Books, 2007.

Benson, Herbert, M.D., with Miriam Z. Klipper. *The Relaxation Response*. New York: Harper Paperbacks, 2000.

Burns, David D., M.D. *Feeling Good: The New Mood Therapy*. New York: Avon, 1999.

Dyer, Wayne W., M.D. *The Power of Intention*. Carlsbad, CA: Hay House, Inc., 2004.

Epstein, Gerald, M.D. *Healing Visualizations: Creating Health Through Imagery*. New York: Bantam, 1989.

Ihnen, Anne, M.A., L.M.H.C., and Carolyn Flynn. *The Complete Idiot's Guide to Mindfulness*. Indianapolis: Alpha Books, 2008.

Kabat-Zinn, Jon, Ph.D. *Full Catastrophe Living*. New York: Delta, 1990.

Naparstek, Belleruth. *Staying Well with Guided Imagery*. New York: Grand Central Publishing, 1995. (She also has multiple guided imagery CDs available.)

Pennebaker, James, Ph.D. *Writing to Heal*. Oakland, CA: New Harbinger Publications, 2004.

Pert, Candace B., Ph.D. *Molecules of Emotion*. New York: Simon & Schuster, 1997.

Rossman, Martin L., M.D. *Guided Imagery for Self-Healing, Second Edition*. Novato, CA: New World Library, 2000.

Sapolsky, Robert M., Ph.D. *Why Zebras Don't Get Ulcers*. New York: Henry Holt and Company, 1998.

Sarno, John, M.D. *The Mindbody Prescription: Healing the Body, Healing the Pain*. New York: Warner Books, 1998.

Sobel, David S., M.D., and Robert Ornstein, Ph.D. *The Healthy Mind Healthy Body Handbook*. New York: Patient Education Media, Inc., 1996.

Williams, J. Mark G., John D. Teasdale, Zindel V. Segal, and Jon Kabat-Zinn. *The Mindful Way Through Depression: Freeing Yourself from Chronic Unhappiness* (with audio CD narrated by Jon Kabat-Zinn). New York: The Guilford Press, 2007.

"Meditations for Relaxation and Stress Reduction," audio CD by Joan Borysenko, Hay House, 2005.

"Practicing the Power of Now: Essential Teachings, Meditations, and Exercises from The Power of Now," audio CD by Eckhart Tolle, 2003.

"Relaxation Body Scan & Guided Imagery for Well-Being," audio CD by Carolyn McManus, P.T., M.S., M.A., 2003.

Chapter 19: The Power of Optimism, Hope, and Laughter

Cousins, Norman. *Anatomy of an Illness as Perceived by the Patient.* New York: W.W. Norton & Company, 1979.

Klein, Allen, and Jeremy Tarcher. *The Healing Power of Humor.* New York: Putnam/Penguin, 1989.

Nahemow, Lucille, Kathleen A. McCluskey-Fawcett, and Paul McGhee, eds. *Humor and Aging.* Academic Press, 1986.

Seligman, Martin, E.P., Ph.D. *Authentic Happiness.* New York: Free Press/Simon & Schuster, 2002.

Vaillant, George, M.D. *Aging Well.* Boston: Little Brown and Co., 2002.

Zander, Rosamund Stone, and Ben Zander. *The Art of Possibility: Transforming Professional and Personal Life.* New York: Penguin 2002.

The Humor Project, www.humorproject.com/about/

Laughter Yoga, www.laughteryoga.org/index.php

Chapter 20: Staying Motivated and Energized to Change

Chopra, Deepak, Ph.D. *The Seven Spiritual Laws of Success.* CA: Amber-Allen Publishing, 1994.

Langer, Ellen, Ph.D. *Mindfulness.* A Merloyd Lawrence Book, Cambridge, MA: Da Capo Press, 1989.

Prochaska, James O., Ph.D., John C. Norcross, Ph.D., and Carlo C. Diclemente, Ph.D. *Changing for Good.* New York: Harper Collins, 1994.

Mastermind Groups, www.imcaz.org/mastermind.html

Chapter 21: Spirituality: The Final Frontier

Chodron, Pema. *When Things Fall Apart: Heart Advice for Difficult Times.* Boston: Shambhala, 2005.

Dossey, Larry, M.D. *Healing Words: The Power of Prayer and the Practice of Medicine.* New York: HarperCollins, 1993.

Katie, Byron. *Loving What Is.* New York: Three Rivers Press, 2003.

Luskin, Fred, Ph.D. *Forgive for Good: A Proven Prescription for Health and Happiness.* New York: HarperCollins, 2002.

Peterson, Christopher, and Martin Seligman. *Character Strengths and Virtues: A Handbook and Classification.* Oxford University Press, 2004.

Tolle, Eckhart. *A New Earth.* New York: Plume/Penguin, 2005.

Boston Medical Center—"New England Centenarian Study," www.bumc.bu.edu/dept/home.aspx?departmentID=361

The University of Georgia College of Public Health, Institute of Gerontology—"Georgia Centenarian Study," www.geron.uga.edu/research/centenarianstudy.php

Index